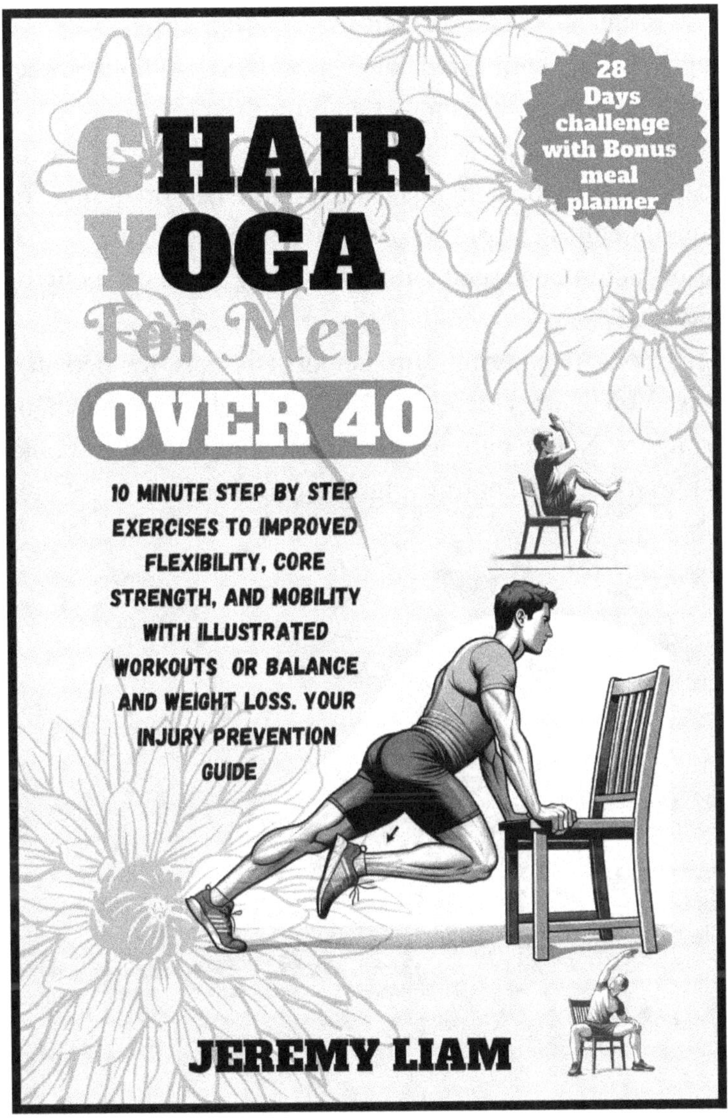

CHAIR YOGA For Men OVER 40

28 Days challenge with Bonus meal planner

10 MINUTE STEP BY STEP EXERCISES TO IMPROVED FLEXIBILITY, CORE STRENGTH, AND MOBILITY WITH ILLUSTRATED WORKOUTS OR BALANCE AND WEIGHT LOSS. YOUR INJURY PREVENTION GUIDE

JEREMY LIAM

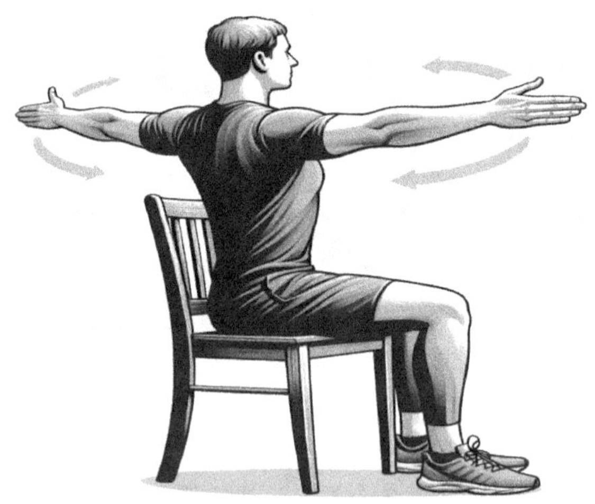

TABLE OF CONTENTS

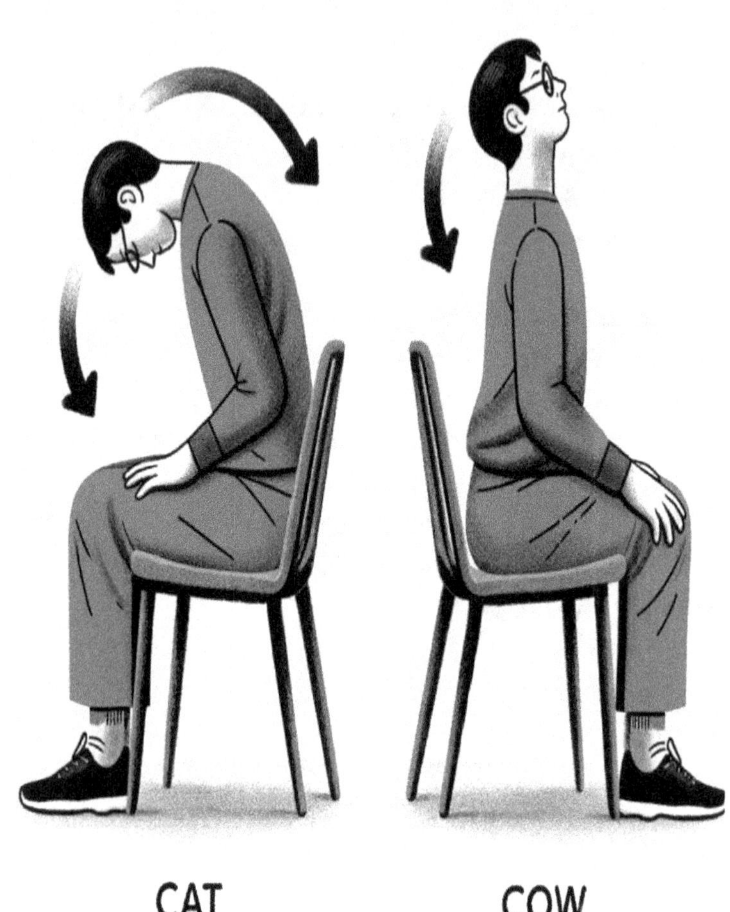

Seated Cat-Cow Stretch

INTRODUCTION

The quest for convenience often leads us down a path of unhealthy lifestyle choices, particularly concerning diet and physical activity. The repercussions of these choices are far-reaching, extending beyond mere physical appearance and impacting our very wellbeing. One of the most significant, yet frequently overlooked, consequences is the heightened risk of injury.

A diet laden with processed foods, high in sugars and unhealthy fats, coupled with a sedentary lifestyle, sets the stage for a myriad of health issues. Poor nutrition weakens the body in several ways. It leads to weight gain, putting excessive stress on bones and joints. The lack of essential nutrients diminishes muscle strength and bone density, making the body more susceptible to injuries.

There was an office worker named Michael. He was a man dedicated to his profession, yet his commitment came at a cost. Hours upon hours spent glued to his screen led Michael to become overweight, struggling with a lack of mobility, poor balance and coordination, weakened core strength, and limited flexibility. Mentally, the toll was evident; the vibrant spirit that once defined him had dimmed under the weight of his physical and mental challenges. Traditional exercises seemed too intense, exacerbating his feelings of inadequacy and further entrenching him in a state of inertia.

It was during this challenging time that our paths crossed. As a fitness instructor specializing in chair yoga, I could see the potential for transformation within Michael. I introduced him to the gentle yet powerful world of chair yoga, a practice that promised to meet him where he was, offering a beacon of hope amidst his struggles.

We embarked on a 28-day challenge, a journey designed not just to alter his physical state but to revitalize his entire being. The chair became his sanctuary, a place from which he could rebuild his strength, regain his flexibility, and restore his mental clarity. Each day, Michael engaged in a series of tailored chair yoga exercises, movements that respected his body's current limitations while gently pushing its boundaries.

The transformation was gradual but profound. With each passing day, Michael's balance improved, his movements became more coordinated, and his core strength solidified. The chair yoga poses, once a challenge, now flowed with an ease that mirrored his growing confidence. But the change wasn't confined to his yoga practice alone.

Alongside the physical exercises, we introduced a meal plan specifically designed to nourish his body and support his journey. The dietary changes complemented his physical efforts, providing the energy he needed to embrace each day's challenges and the nutrients essential for his body's rejuvenation.

The 28-day challenge was more than a test of physical endurance; it was a holistic journey that transformed Michael's perspective on health and wellness. The chair, once a symbol of his sedentary lifestyle, had become a tool for empowerment. Michael's dedication to the challenge was unwavering, and with each day, the benefits multiplied, extending beyond the physical realm and permeating every aspect of his life.

As we reached the conclusion of the challenge, the transformation was undeniable. Michael was not only stronger and more flexible physically, but he had also rediscovered a mental resilience that had long been buried under the demands of his office life. The journey through chair yoga had rekindled his inner strength, illuminated a path to wellness, and redefined his understanding of what it means to be truly healthy.

Michael's story is a testament to the transformative power of chair yoga, a reminder that wellness is a holistic journey that harmonizes the body, mind, and spirit. It's a story of renewal, a narrative that echoes the potential within each of us to overcome our limitations and embrace a life of balance, strength, and vitality. As Michael's instructor, witnessing his journey was not just a privilege but a profound reminder of the life-changing impact of empathy, dedication, and the gentle power of chair yoga.

As a gym instructor, my journey has always been centered around movement, strength, and the pursuit of physical wellness. Over the years, I've witnessed countless transformations, not just in body, but in spirit and mind. Yet, one aspect that often went unnoticed, especially among men over 40, was the subtle yet powerful art of chair yoga. This practice, often overshadowed by more vigorous forms of exercise, holds a special place in my heart and in the lives of those I've had the privilege to guide.

Chair yoga, in its essence, is a practice that embodies accessibility, mindfulness, and a gentle path to fitness, tailored especially for those who might find traditional yoga or high-impact workouts challenging. As I ventured deeper into this discipline, I discovered a world where fitness was not just about how much one could lift or how fast one could run, but about balance, flexibility, and a harmony between body and mind.

In my years of teaching, I noticed a common trend among men over 40. They came to me with stories of past injuries, chronic pain, or simply a sense of intimidation by the high-energy atmosphere of typical gym sessions. They sought something that could offer them health benefits without the strain, something that was gentle yet effective. This is where chair yoga emerged not just as an exercise, but as a holistic solution.

The beauty of chair yoga lies in its simplicity and adaptability. A chair, an everyday object, becomes a tool for transformation. In my sessions, I've seen men who had given up on the idea of flexibility, regain their range of motion. I've witnessed those who struggled with balance, find a new sense of stability. Weight loss, core strength, improved posture, and injury prevention – all these benefits flowed naturally from regular practice.

Chair yoga goes beyond physical wellness. It's a gateway to mental clarity and emotional balance. In a world where stress is a constant, this practice offers a sanctuary. The breathing techniques and mindful movements are not just exercises; they are invitations to a more centered, peaceful state of being.

In this book, I invite you on a journey. It's a journey that starts with a simple chair and an open mind. Whether you're dealing with the physical challenges that come with age, looking to enhance your fitness routine, or seeking a new path to mental well-being, chair yoga has something to offer. Through my experiences and the wisdom gleaned from years of teaching, I'll guide you through each step, helping you discover a stronger, more flexible, and more balanced version of yourself.

CHAPTER 1: THE POWER OF CHAIR YOGA

As a gym instructor with years of experience in guiding people towards their fitness goals, I have come to appreciate the subtle yet profound power of chair yoga, especially for those in the over-40 age bracket. This practice, often underestimated, unfolds its true potential when approached with an open mind and heart.

Chair yoga is not just about adapting traditional yoga poses to a seated position; it's about redefining what fitness and well-being mean as we age. In my journey as an instructor, I've seen men walk into the gym, their faces etched with the reluctance that comes from past injuries or the intimidation of high-intensity workouts. They often feel disconnected from their bodies, as if flexibility and strength are relics of their youth. But through chair yoga, I've witnessed remarkable transformations.

The power of chair yoga lies in its accessibility. A chair, a simple piece of furniture, becomes an anchor, a stabilizing force that allows these men to explore movements they thought were no longer within their reach. Each session becomes an exploration, a gentle push against the boundaries of what they believe is possible.

What truly sets chair yoga apart is its holistic approach. It's not just about the physical act of moving; it's a dance of breath and body, a practice that intertwines the physical with the mental and emotional. In my classes, as we move through each pose, there's a palpable shift in the room. The initial hesitancy gives way to a rhythm, a flow that enlivens not just the body, but also the spirit.

Chair yoga offers a path to regain what many men over 40 feel they have lost. Balance, which starts to wane with age, is nurtured and strengthened. The slow, controlled movements coupled with deep, mindful breathing enhance flexibility and core strength, all while minimizing the risk of injury. It's not uncommon to see a newfound sense of confidence and vitality in my clients as they progress.

But perhaps the most profound aspect of chair yoga is its impact on mental health. In a world brimming with stress and anxiety, chair yoga offers a sanctuary of calm. The focus on breathwork and mindful movement fosters a sense of inner peace, a quieting of the mind that many find elusive in their daily lives.

Through my experience as a gym instructor, I have come to see chair yoga not just as an exercise routine, but as a journey towards holistic health and wellness. It's a journey of rediscovering one's body, of finding balance and peace, and of redefining what it means to age gracefully and healthily. Chair yoga, in its essence, is a testament to the enduring strength and adaptability of the human body and spirit.

<u>What is chair yoga?</u>

I've always been drawn to the transformative power of exercise. But it was my encounter with chair yoga that truly expanded my understanding of what fitness and wellness could mean, especially for those over 40. Chair yoga, often perceived as a simplified form of traditional yoga, is in fact a deeply effective and accessible discipline that opens new avenues of health and vitality.

At its core, chair yoga is about adaptability and accessibility. It takes the ancient practice of yoga and modifies it to be performed with the aid of a chair, making it suitable for individuals who might face limitations with mobility, balance, or endurance. This simple adaptation opens the doors of yoga to a much wider audience, particularly benefiting those who might feel excluded from conventional exercise routines.

In my classes, chair yoga begins as a gentle the world of yoga. We use the chair not just as a prop, but as a companion in the journey towards better health. It offers support, stability, and a sense of safety, allowing practitioners to explore movements and poses without the fear of strain or injury. This sense of security is crucial, especially for men over 40 who may be dealing with the physical changes that come with age.

But chair yoga is more than just a series of seated poses. It's a holistic practice that integrates the body, mind, and spirit. As a gym instructor, I've seen firsthand how chair yoga can positively impact not just physical health, but also mental and emotional well-being. The practice encourages mindfulness and breath awareness, creating a meditative state that reduces stress and enhances mental clarity.

One of the most remarkable aspects of chair yoga is its ability to be both gentle and challenging. While it provides a safe way to increase flexibility, strengthen muscles, and improve posture, it also challenges practitioners to push their limits within a safe boundary. It's about finding one's edge and gently expanding it, leading to gradual but significant improvements in overall fitness and well-being.

Through my experience, I've come to see chair yoga not just as a series of exercises, but as a journey. It's a path that embraces the changes in our bodies as we age, offering a way to maintain and even enhance our physical and mental health. It's a practice that acknowledges and respects limitations, while also celebrating progress and growth. Chair yoga, in essence, is a testament to the resilience and adaptability of the human body and spirit, a practice that truly embodies the philosophy that fitness is for everyone, at every stage of life.

How chair yoga made a difference

Chair yoga has not just been another exercise option; it has emerged as a transformative practice, redefining the boundaries of what fitness means for an aging population.

The difference chair yoga has made is profound and multifaceted. At its most basic, it provides a safe, low-impact form of exercise, crucial for men dealing with the physical constraints of age. The chair, a simple and unassuming piece of equipment, becomes a powerful tool for stability and support. This enables individuals who might otherwise shy away from exercise due to fear of injury or discomfort to engage in physical activity confidently.

But the impact of chair yoga goes far beyond mere physical fitness. It has become a conduit for restoring and maintaining mobility, an aspect of health that is often taken for granted until it begins to decline. Through carefully designed sequences and poses, my clients have seen remarkable improvements in their flexibility and range of motion. I've witnessed men who were initially unable to perform basic movements without discomfort gradually regain a level of mobility that they thought they had lost forever.

Moreover, chair yoga transcends physical wellness and touches upon the mental and emotional aspects of health. In my classes, I've observed how the practice fosters a sense of mental clarity and emotional balance. The focus on mindful movements and breathing creates a meditative state that alleviates stress and promotes a sense of inner peace. This mental and emotional upliftment is particularly beneficial for men over 40, who often grapple with the stresses and pressures of mid-life.

One of the most gratifying aspects of incorporating chair yoga into my teachings has been witnessing the community it builds. Unlike traditional gym environments that can sometimes feel competitive and intimidating, chair yoga fosters a sense of camaraderie and support among its practitioners. It's a space where individuals come together, not just to improve their own health, but to encourage and uplift each other.

Chair yoga, in my experience, has been more than just an addition to a fitness regime; it has been a life-changing practice for many of my clients. It has allowed them to redefine their relationship with their bodies, to embrace aging with grace and strength, and to understand that fitness and wellness are achievable and sustainable at any age. The difference it has made is not just in the physical transformations I've seen, but in the renewed sense of vitality and the joy of movement it has brought into the lives of those I instruct.

Core Principles of Yoga and Their Adaptation to Chair Yoga

As a gym instructor deeply immersed in the world of fitness, my exploration into yoga and its adaptation into chair yoga has been a journey of discovery and enlightenment. Yoga, with its rich heritage, extends far beyond mere physical postures. It's a discipline that encompasses a holistic approach to wellbeing, integrating the mind, body, and spirit. In translating these core principles into chair yoga, especially for my clients over 40, I've seen a remarkable synergy between ancient wisdom and modern practicality.

One of the foundational principles of yoga is 'Ahimsa', which means non-harm. This principle is pivotal in chair yoga, where the emphasis is on gentle movements that respect the body's limitations and needs. In my classes, this translates to a practice that encourages mindfulness and self-awareness, allowing each individual to honor their body's unique capacities and avoid injury. This approach is particularly resonant for men over 40, who often face the challenges of age-related physical changes.

Another key element of yoga is 'Pranayama', or breath control. In chair yoga, breath becomes the anchor of the practice, guiding each movement and fostering a deep connection between the body and mind. Through focused breathing techniques, my clients have experienced improved mental clarity, reduced stress levels, and an enhanced sense of inner peace. This aspect of yoga, adapted to a seated practice, has been instrumental in creating a holistic fitness experience.

The principle of 'Dhyana', or meditation, also finds its place in chair yoga. Each session becomes an opportunity for stillness and reflection. In the midst of their busy lives, this practice offers my clients a moment of tranquility, where they can cultivate mindfulness and a deeper sense of self-awareness. This meditative aspect of chair yoga has proven invaluable for mental and emotional wellbeing, especially for those navigating the complexities of mid-life.

Moreover, the concept of 'Asana', or posture, in traditional yoga, is creatively adapted in chair yoga. The chair aids in modifying poses, making them accessible and beneficial for those who might struggle with balance or flexibility. This adaptation ensures that the physical benefits of yoga, such as improved strength, flexibility, and balance, are within reach for everyone, regardless of their physical condition.

In integrating these core principles of yoga into chair yoga, I've witnessed a beautiful transformation in my clients. They've embraced a practice that not only enhances their physical health but also nourishes their mental and emotional wellbeing. As a gym instructor, facilitating this journey has been a fulfilling experience, reinforcing the timeless relevance of yoga's principles and their adaptability to the needs of modern life. Chair yoga, in essence, is a testament to the universality of yoga and its capacity to enrich lives, regardless of age or physical ability.

Breathwork and Mindfulness Techniques

I've always emphasized the importance of physical fitness. However, the introduction of breathwork and mindfulness techniques into my sessions has opened a new dimension, not only for me but for the many individuals I guide, especially those over 40. These techniques, integral to the practice of chair yoga, have become a cornerstone of our routines, offering benefits that extend well beyond the physical.

Breathwork, or the conscious control of breathing, is more than just a means to enhance physical performance; it's a powerful tool for mental and emotional regulation. In chair yoga, we use various breathing techniques to deepen the connection between the body and mind. These techniques range from simple deep breathing to more structured practices like the 'Ujjayi' breath, known for its calming and grounding effects. Through breathwork, my clients have learned to manage stress, reduce anxiety, and attain a sense of inner calm. This is particularly beneficial for men over 40, who often juggle the demands of career, family, and personal health.

Incorporating mindfulness into our chair yoga sessions has further enriched the experience. Mindfulness, the practice of being fully present and engaged in the moment, has transformed how we approach each movement and pose. It encourages a heightened awareness of the body, fostering a deeper understanding of its capabilities and limitations. This awareness is crucial for preventing injuries and creating a more attuned and respectful relationship with one's own body.

Moreover, mindfulness extends beyond physical awareness. It encompasses an awareness of one's thoughts and emotions, fostering a non-judgmental and compassionate attitude towards oneself. For many of my clients, this aspect of chair yoga has been life-changing. In a world where constant stimulation and stress are the norms, the ability to find a quiet, centered space within oneself is invaluable.

The combined practice of breathwork and mindfulness has not only enhanced the physical benefits of chair yoga but has also provided a path to holistic well-being. My clients have reported improved sleep, better concentration, and an overall sense of well-being that they carry with them long after the class ends.

As a gym instructor, incorporating these techniques into my teaching has been a profoundly rewarding experience. It has allowed me to offer a more holistic approach to fitness, one that addresses the needs of the body, mind, and spirit. Breathwork and mindfulness are not just exercises; they are tools for living a more balanced, healthy, and fulfilling life, especially critical as we navigate the complexities of mid-life and beyond.

Mental and emotional merit of chair yoga

In my role as a gym instructor, I have long been an advocate for the physical benefits of exercise. However, my foray into chair yoga has shed light on a vital aspect often overshadowed in traditional fitness routines: the mental and emotional merits. Chair yoga, while physically engaging, offers profound mental and emotional benefits, especially significant for individuals over 40, a demographic I frequently work with.

The beauty of chair yoga lies not just in its physical accessibility but in its power to soothe and strengthen the mind and spirit. In our fast-paced world, stress, anxiety, and emotional turmoil are commonplace, especially as one navigates the challenges of mid-life. Chair yoga offers a sanctuary, a rare space where mental and emotional wellness is prioritized.

The practice begins with the breath, the bridge between the body and mind. In chair yoga, we focus on deep, mindful breathing, which has a calming effect on the nervous system. This simple yet powerful technique helps in reducing stress and anxiety, promoting a sense of tranquility. As a gym instructor, I've seen firsthand how this focus on breathwork can transform a state of mental chaos into one of calm and clarity.

The poses and movements in chair yoga, while gentle, require concentration and presence, fostering a state of mindfulness. This mindfulness - the practice of being fully engaged in the present moment - has been a revelation for many of my clients. It teaches them to observe their thoughts and emotions without judgment, creating a space of self-awareness and self-compassion. In a culture that often prioritizes physical appearance and performance over mental health, this aspect of chair yoga offers a refreshing and much-needed shift in focus.

Furthermore, the communal aspect of chair yoga fosters a sense of connection and belonging. Many of my clients over 40 have expressed feelings of isolation or disconnection. The shared experience of chair yoga creates a supportive community where emotions and experiences can be shared and validated. This sense of community is instrumental in enhancing emotional well-being.

The mental and emotional merits of chair yoga extend beyond the session. My clients often report a carryover effect into their daily lives. They find themselves more patient, less reactive, and more emotionally balanced. They develop tools to manage stress and face challenges with a calmer, more centered approach.

Incorporating chair yoga into my teaching repertoire has thus been a profoundly fulfilling experience. It has allowed me to offer a holistic approach to wellness, addressing not just the physical but also the mental and emotional needs of my clients. In a world that often neglects these aspects of health, chair yoga stands as a testament to the importance of nurturing the mind and spirit, as much as the body.

Nutrition Tips to Complement Your Yoga Practice

I've come to understand the inseparable relationship between nutrition and exercise. This understanding deepened as I delved into the world of chair yoga, especially in guiding men over 40. I've learned that while chair yoga offers immense physical and mental benefits, these can be significantly enhanced with the right nutritional approach. Good nutrition is not just about feeding the body; it's about nourishing the whole self, complementing the holistic nature of yoga.

Nutrition, in the context of chair yoga, goes beyond the typical fitness diet focused solely on macros and calories. It's about embracing a way of eating that supports flexibility, energy, and mental clarity – all key components of a successful yoga practice. The first step is hydration. Proper hydration is crucial, as even mild dehydration can affect flexibility and concentration. I encourage my clients to drink water throughout the day, especially before and after their yoga sessions.

The next aspect is balance. A balanced diet, rich in whole foods, provides the energy and nutrients needed to support a yoga practice. I often advise my clients to focus on a variety of fruits, vegetables, whole grains, lean proteins, and healthy fats. This variety ensures a broad spectrum of essential vitamins and minerals, aiding in muscle recovery, joint health, and overall vitality.

Another key element is timing. The timing of meals in relation to yoga practice is important. A heavy meal just before yoga can be uncomfortable, while practicing on an empty stomach might lead to lack of energy and concentration. A light snack, preferably something easy to digest like a piece of fruit or a small yogurt, can be ideal before a session. Post-yoga, a balanced meal helps in recovery and refueling the body.

Mindful eating also forms a crucial part of this nutritional approach. Just as chair yoga encourages mindfulness in movement, mindful eating emphasizes being present and attentive to the experience of eating. This practice not only enhances the enjoyment of food but also encourages a healthier relationship with eating, tuning into hunger cues and satiety signals.

Through my experience as a gym instructor, integrating nutrition tips into chair yoga practice has been rewarding. It has allowed me to provide a more comprehensive wellness approach, emphasizing that taking care of the body through nutrition is as important as the physical practice of yoga itself. This approach not only supports the physical aspects of yoga but also aligns with its holistic philosophy, leading to a more balanced and fulfilling lifestyle.

Lifestyle Changes for Sustainable Weight Loss

In my years as a gym instructor, guiding people through their fitness journeys, I've learned that sustainable weight loss is much more than just a series of workouts or diet plans. It's about lifestyle changes, small yet significant shifts in daily habits that create a lasting impact. This understanding has been especially crucial in my work with men over

40, where I've integrated chair yoga as a part of their fitness regime.

The key to sustainable weight loss, I've found, lies in a holistic approach that combines physical activity with broader lifestyle adjustments. Chair yoga plays a pivotal role here, not just as a form of exercise, but as a catalyst for a healthier, more balanced way of living. It's not about drastic, short-term fixes, but about creating a sustainable, enjoyable way of life that naturally supports weight management.

Firstly, incorporating regular physical activity is crucial, and chair yoga offers an accessible and enjoyable way to do this. Its low-impact, gentle nature makes it a perfect fit for those who might find traditional workouts daunting or too strenuous. However, the journey doesn't stop at exercise. It extends into other areas of life, such as nutrition, sleep, and stress management.

One of the most significant lifestyle changes I advocate for is in the realm of nutrition. Adopting a balanced diet, rich in whole foods, and mindful eating practices greatly supports weight loss. It's not about severe restriction or fad diets; instead, it's about learning to listen to the body and nourish it properly. This approach not only aids in weight loss but also enhances the overall quality of life.

Sleep is another critical factor. Good quality sleep has a direct impact on weight management. In my sessions, I often incorporate relaxation and breathing techniques from chair yoga to help improve sleep quality. These techniques help in reducing stress, which is another crucial aspect. Chronic stress can lead to weight gain, particularly around the midsection, a common concern for men over 40. Chair yoga, with its emphasis on mindfulness and relaxation, offers an effective way to manage stress.

Finally, building a supportive community is invaluable. Whether it's family, friends, or fellow yoga practitioners, having a network of support fosters motivation and accountability.

In my experience, these lifestyle changes, when combined with regular chair yoga practice, create a powerful formula for sustainable weight loss. It's not just about shedding pounds; it's about building a lifestyle that naturally supports a healthy weight and overall well-being. This approach has not only helped my clients lose weight but also find a more balanced, fulfilling way of living.

Everyday Tips for Maintaining Good Posture

In my career as a gym instructor, one of the most common concerns among my clients, especially those over 40, is maintaining good posture. The modern lifestyle, often characterized by long hours sitting at desks or hunched over smartphones, has made posture-related issues increasingly prevalent. As someone deeply involved in fitness and well-being, I've learned that maintaining good posture is not just about looking confident; it's about promoting overall health and preventing a myriad of musculoskeletal problems.

My foray into chair yoga has been instrumental in addressing this issue. Chair yoga not only helps in strengthening the muscles necessary for good posture but also heightened body awareness, which is crucial for correcting postural habits. However, maintaining good posture extends beyond the confines of a yoga session. It's about small, consistent changes in daily habits that make a significant difference.

One of the everyday tips I emphasize is being mindful of posture while sitting. In a world dominated by desk jobs, the way we sit for hours plays a crucial role in our spinal health. I encourage my clients to choose chairs that support the natural curve of the spine, to keep their feet flat on the floor, and to avoid crossing their legs. Simple adjustments such as ensuring the computer screen is at eye level can significantly reduce the strain on the neck and shoulders.

Another key aspect is staying active. Prolonged periods of sitting can lead to muscle stiffness and weaken the postural muscles. I advise incorporating short, frequent breaks into the daily routine to stretch and walk around. Even simple stretches or chair yoga poses at the desk can be immensely beneficial.

Strengthening the core is another vital component of maintaining good posture. A strong core supports the spine, reducing the likelihood of slouching and back pain. Chair yoga includes several poses that enhance core strength, and these can be easily practiced even while at work.

Furthermore, being conscious of posture while walking and standing is equally important. I often suggest practicing standing tall, with shoulders relaxed and aligned over the hips, imagining a string pulling from the top of the head towards the ceiling. This visualization can help in maintaining an upright, balanced posture.

Lastly, the role of a good night's sleep in posture cannot be overstated. Using a supportive mattress and pillow can help maintain the spine's natural alignment, contributing to better posture during waking hours.

In my experience, these everyday tips, coupled with regular chair yoga practice, have been effective in helping my clients improve their posture. It's a holistic approach, integrating mindful practices, physical activity, and lifestyle adjustments to foster not just better posture, but overall health and well-being.

<u>Tips for preventing falls and injuries</u>

I've come to realize the importance of preventing falls and injuries, especially in individuals over 40. This age group is often at a higher risk due to factors like decreased muscle strength, balance issues, and slower reflexes. As someone dedicated to promoting health and fitness, I've focused on imparting knowledge and techniques that help in reducing this risk, integrating the principles I've learned through chair yoga and general fitness training.

One of the key aspects of preventing falls is developing balance and stability. In chair yoga, many of the poses are designed to enhance these attributes. While the chair provides support, it also allows for the safe practice of balance-improving exercises. However, the journey to preventing falls extends beyond the yoga mat or gym floor. It's about incorporating balance and coordination exercises into daily routines, making it a habit to challenge and enhance these skills regularly.

Strength training, particularly of the lower body, plays a crucial role in fall prevention. Stronger muscles, especially in the legs and core, provide better support for the body, improving stability and reducing the likelihood of falls. In my sessions, I emphasize exercises that strengthen these areas, ensuring that they are suitable for all fitness levels, with a focus on safety and gradual progression.

Another crucial factor is environmental awareness. Many falls occur due to hazards like slippery floors, uneven surfaces, or poor lighting. I advise my clients to be mindful of their surroundings, both at home and while out. Simple measures like using non-slip mats, ensuring good lighting, and wearing appropriate footwear can significantly reduce the risk of falls.

Additionally, educating about proper body mechanics is vital. Understanding how to move correctly, how to lift objects without straining the back, and how to navigate through spaces safely is essential. This education, combined with exercises that enhance flexibility and range of motion, contributes to a better awareness of body positioning, further aiding in injury prevention.

Nutrition and hydration also play a role in preventing falls. A diet rich in calcium and vitamin D supports bone health, while adequate hydration ensures good muscle function. I encourage a balanced diet and regular fluid intake as part of a comprehensive approach to fall prevention.

Lastly, regular health check-ups, including vision and hearing tests, are important. These aspects, often overlooked, can significantly impact balance and spatial awareness.

Integrating these tips into my clients' routines has led to a noticeable decrease in the frequency of falls and related injuries. It's about creating a holistic approach that combines exercise, environmental adjustments, and lifestyle changes, all aimed at ensuring a safer, more stable, and healthier life.

<u>Yoga for common age related concerns</u>

I've often encountered clients, particularly those over 40, grappling with common age-related concerns. These range from reduced flexibility and joint pain to stress and sleep disturbances. My exploration into yoga, especially chair yoga, has provided invaluable tools to address these issues. Yoga, with its holistic approach, offers much more than physical exercise – it presents a pathway to manage and alleviate the challenges that come with aging.

One of the most prevalent issues I see in my older clients is reduced flexibility and stiffness in the joints. Yoga, with its emphasis on gentle stretching and movement, has proven to be a game changer. Chair yoga, in particular, makes these benefits accessible to those who might find traditional yoga poses challenging. The slow, controlled movements help in gradually increasing the range of motion, reducing stiffness, and enhancing flexibility. This improvement in flexibility not only aids in day-to-day activities but also plays a significant role in injury prevention.

Joint pain, often a result of conditions like arthritis, is another common concern. Yoga's low-impact nature makes it an ideal exercise for those suffering from joint pain. The gentle poses and stretches, supported by the chair, allow for movement without putting undue stress on the joints. Moreover, yoga's focus on breathwork and mindfulness offers an added advantage in managing pain perception, helping clients cope better with chronic pain.

Stress and anxiety are also significant issues, particularly in the fast-paced lives many lead. Yoga's meditative aspect, with deep breathing and mindfulness practices, has a profoundly calming effect on the mind. It helps in reducing cortisol levels, the stress hormone, promoting a sense of relaxation and well-being. I've seen clients who practice yoga regularly report better stress management and an overall improved quality of life.

Sleep disturbances, often more frequent as one ages, can also be alleviated through yoga. The relaxation techniques and breathing exercises practiced in yoga have been shown to improve sleep quality. Clients often tell me how incorporating yoga into their routine has helped them achieve a deeper, more restful sleep.

From my experience, integrating yoga into fitness routines for those over 40 has not only addressed specific age-related concerns but also enhanced overall health and well-being. It's a testament to yoga's adaptability and its profound impact on managing the challenges of aging.

Who should practice and who should avoid the chair yoga

I've had the privilege of introducing various groups of people to chair yoga. This gentle form of exercise, which adapts traditional yoga poses for a seated or standing position using a chair for support, has been a revelation for many. Its inclusivity and adaptability make it suitable for a wide range of individuals, but like any exercise regime, it's important to understand who stands to benefit most from it and who might need to approach it with caution or seek alternative options.

Chair yoga is particularly beneficial for those who are new to yoga or exercise in general. Its gentle approach makes it an excellent starting point for individuals who are older, particularly those over 40, who might be dealing with the natural physical changes that come with aging. It's also ideal for people who spend a lot of time sitting or have limited mobility due to various reasons such as chronic health conditions, recovery from surgery, or physical disabilities. The accessibility of chair yoga allows these individuals to engage in physical activity without the fear of strain or injury.

Furthermore, chair yoga is a boon for those who spend long hours at a desk. Office workers and professionals can incorporate chair yoga into their daily routine to alleviate the stiffness and discomfort that comes from prolonged sitting. It's a great way to introduce movement and stretching into a sedentary lifestyle, offering benefits like improved posture, enhanced flexibility, and reduced stress.

However, there are also individuals who should approach chair yoga with caution or may need to avoid it altogether. People with certain health conditions, such as severe osteoporosis, advanced heart diseases, or those who have recently undergone surgery, should consult their healthcare provider before beginning a chair yoga practice. It's crucial that these individuals get a go-ahead from a medical professional to ensure that the poses and movements in chair yoga are safe for their specific health conditions.

Additionally, those who are looking for a high-intensity, calorie-burning workout might find chair yoga less fulfilling in terms of their fitness goals. While chair yoga does improve strength, flexibility, and balance, it is inherently a low-impact and gentle form of exercise.

The beauty of chair yoga lies in its adaptability. With appropriate modifications and guidance, it can be tailored to suit the needs of most individuals, making it a versatile tool in the realm of fitness and wellness. It stands as a testament to the philosophy that exercise, in any form, should be inclusive and accessible to all.

How to keep up when things get hard

One of the most common challenges my clients face is staying motivated, especially when the going gets tough. Whether it's a fitness plateau, a lack of visible progress, or simply the everyday demands of life, these hurdles can sometimes feel insurmountable. Over the years, I've gathered insights and strategies to help keep motivation alive, even in the toughest of times.

Firstly, I've learned the importance of setting realistic and achievable goals. In the initial burst of enthusiasm, it's easy to aim high, but unrealistic goals can quickly become demotivating when they are not met. I encourage my clients to set smaller, incremental targets that add up to their larger goal. This approach brings a sense of accomplishment and progress, keeping the motivation high.

Another key aspect is finding the right balance. Often, people dive into intense workout routines or strict diets, which are not sustainable in the long run. I advise a more balanced approach, integrating exercise into daily life in a way that is enjoyable and manageable. It could be as simple as choosing chair yoga over high-intensity workouts on days when energy levels are low, or opting for a nutritious meal that's also satisfying rather than a restrictive diet.

I also emphasize the power of routine. Building a consistent exercise schedule helps in making fitness a part of everyday life. However, it's important to remain flexible and adapt when necessary. Life can be unpredictable, and being too rigid with routines can lead to frustration. It's about finding that sweet spot where exercise becomes a regular, enjoyable part of life, without feeling like a chore.

Support systems play a crucial role as well. Whether it's a workout buddy, a supportive family member, or a fitness community, having people who understand and support your journey can make a significant difference. They can provide encouragement, share in the struggles, and celebrate the victories, big or small.

Lastly, I always remind my clients to be kind to themselves. There will be days when motivation is low, and that's okay. It's important to acknowledge that fitness journeys are not linear. There will be ups and downs, and learning to navigate these with self-compassion and resilience is key.

In my journey as an instructor, guiding people through these challenges has been as rewarding as celebrating their successes. It's about fostering a mindset that sees challenges as part of the journey, learning to adapt and stay the course even when things get hard.

CHAPTER 2: SETTING UP YOUR PRACTICE SPACE

Setting up a practice space for chair yoga or any fitness routine is an important step in creating an environment that is conducive to a focused and effective workout. Drawing from my experience as a gym instructor, I've learned that the right space can significantly enhance the quality of your practice. Here are some key considerations for setting up your practice space:

1. Choose the Right Location: Select a space that is quiet, comfortable, and free from distractions. It doesn't have to be large, but it should be enough for you to move freely. An area that receives natural light and has good ventilation is ideal.

2. Ensure Enough Space: Make sure there's enough room to extend your arms and legs fully in all directions. A good rule of thumb is to have at least an arm's length of space around your chair.

3. Select an Appropriate Chair: The chair you use should be sturdy and comfortable. Avoid chairs with wheels or armrests, as they can restrict movement or pose a safety risk. The chair should be of a height where your feet can rest flat on the ground while seated.

4. Invest in a Good Mat: If you're practicing on a hard surface, consider using a yoga mat for additional grip and cushioning. This is especially helpful for any standing poses or floor work.

5. Minimize Clutter: Keep the area around your practice space free of clutter. A clean and organized space helps in maintaining focus and reduces the risk of accidents.

6. Create a Calming Atmosphere: Consider elements that enhance the tranquility of your space. This could be anything from soft lighting, such as candles or dimmable lamps, to playing gentle background music or sounds of nature.

7. Keep Essential Props Handy: Depending on your routine, you might need props like yoga blocks,

straps, or cushions. Keep these within easy reach but out of the way to avoid tripping over them.

8. Personalize Your Space: Add personal touches that make the space inviting and motivating. This could be inspirational quotes, a small plant, or any item that brings you joy and calmness.

Remember, your practice space is your sanctuary. It should be a place where you feel relaxed, focused, and motivated to practice. The effort you put into setting up this space can significantly enhance your overall experience and commitment to your fitness routine.

Essential Equipment: The Right Chair and Accessories

In chair yoga, as in any fitness practice, having the right equipment is crucial for both effectiveness and safety. Based on my experience as a gym instructor, here are the essentials for chair yoga, focusing on the right chair and necessary accessories:

1. The Right Chair:
   - Stability: Choose a chair that is sturdy and stable. It should not have wheels, as they can cause unwanted movement.
   - Size and Height: The chair should be of appropriate height so your feet can rest flat on the floor, and your knees are at a right angle. This alignment is crucial for safety and effectiveness.
   - No Armrests: Ideally, the chair should be without armrests. Armrests can restrict movement during certain yoga poses.

2. Yoga Mat:
   - A yoga mat provides a non-slip surface, which is especially important for any standing poses or floor work you might incorporate alongside chair yoga.

3. Cushions or Blocks:
   - These can be used to ensure proper alignment and to make certain poses more comfortable. For instance, a cushion can be placed on the chair for added comfort or support.

4. Yoga Straps:

- Straps are helpful for those with limited flexibility. They can be used to safely achieve certain positions, like leg stretches, without straining.

5. Resistance Bands:

- These can be incorporated for added strength training. They are useful for exercises targeting arm and leg muscles.

6. Towels or Blankets:

- Useful for providing extra cushioning or support as needed. A folded blanket can be placed on the yoga mat for knee support, or a towel can be used to wipe away sweat.

7. Comfortable Clothing:

- Wear clothing that allows for a full range of motion and is breathable. Avoid very loose clothing as it might get caught or obstruct view of alignment.

8. Water Bottle:

- Hydration is key, even in less intense forms of exercise like chair yoga.

Remember, while these items can enhance your practice, the most important thing is your approach. Listen to your body, respect its limits, and use these tools to aid in your practice, not to push beyond what feels safe and comfortable.

Safe practices guidelines

Ensuring safety during any fitness routine, including chair yoga, is paramount. Based on my experience as a gym instructor, I recommend the following safe practice guidelines:

1. Right Equipment: Use a sturdy chair without wheels, and ensure your equipment (like mats, straps, or blocks) is in good condition and suitable for your practice.

2. Warm-Up: Always begin with a warm-up to prepare your muscles and joints. Gentle stretching and basic movements can help reduce the risk of injury.

3. Be Aware of Your Body: Listen to your body and be mindful of any pain or discomfort. If a pose or movement feels painful, stop immediately. It's crucial to differentiate between a good stretch and pain.

4. Maintain Proper Alignment: Focus on keeping your body properly aligned to avoid strain. If you're unsure about a pose, it's better to err on the side of caution.

5. Don't Rush: Move into and out of poses slowly and with control. Avoid jerky or rapid movements that can lead to loss of balance or strain.

6. Stay Hydrated: Drink water before, during, and after your practice to stay hydrated, especially if you're incorporating more vigorous movements.

7. Know Your Limits: Recognize and respect your physical limits. Don't push too hard or try advanced poses if you're not ready.

8. Use Props When Needed: Don't hesitate to use props like cushions, blocks, or straps for support and

to ensure proper form, especially if you have limited flexibility or balance issues.

9. Focus on Breathing: Proper breathing is not only calming but also helps in maintaining focus and preventing strain. Breathe normally throughout your practice, and don't hold your breath.

10. Cool Down: End your session with a cool-down period. Gentle stretches or relaxation techniques can help your body transition out of the practice.

11. Consult Healthcare Providers: If you have any existing health conditions, injuries, or concerns, consult with a healthcare provider before starting or modifying your exercise routine.

12. Regular Practice: Consistency is key. Regular practice helps your body gradually adapt and reduces the risk of injury.

Remember, the goal of chair yoga is to improve your health and well-being, not to compete or compare. Each person's body is unique, and so is their yoga journey. Take it at your own pace and enjoy the process.

CHAPTER 3: WARMUP EXERCISES

Neck Stretches

Neck stretches are vital in any fitness routine, particularly beneficial for those who spend a lot of time sitting or in static postures. These stretches can alleviate neck stiffness, improve flexibility, and help reduce the risk of neck-related discomfort.

Instructions for Neck Stretches

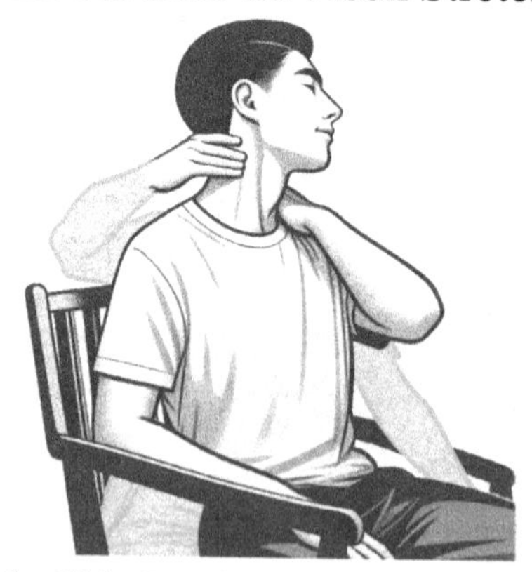

1. Side Neck Stretch:

- Sit upright in a chair, feet flat on the ground.
- Gently tilt your head to the right, bringing your ear towards the shoulder.
- Keep your left shoulder down and relaxed.
- For a deeper stretch, gently press down on your head with your right hand.
- Hold the stretch for 15-30 seconds.
- Return to the center and repeat on the left side.

2. Forward Neck Stretch:
- Sit upright and slowly tilt your chin towards your chest.
- Touch the back of your head with your hands while interlacing your fingers.
- Gently apply pressure, enhancing the stretch in the back of your neck.
- Hold for 15-30 seconds, then release.

3. Backward Neck Stretch:
- Sit upright, place your hands on your hips.
- Look up towards the ceiling with a slight backward tilt of your head.
- Hold for 15-30 seconds, then return to the neutral position.

Number of Sets and Repetitions

- • - Perform each stretch 2-3 times.
- • - Repeat the sequence 1-2 times a day, especially if you spend long periods sitting.
- •

Remember, while performing these stretches, you should feel a gentle pull, but no pain. If you experience any discomfort, reduce the intensity or discontinue the stretch. Regular practice can significantly improve neck flexibility and reduce discomfort.

Shoulder Rolls

Shoulder Rolls are a fundamental exercise for relieving tension and improving mobility in the shoulder area. As a gym instructor, I often recommend this exercise to individuals who experience stiffness or discomfort due to prolonged sitting, repetitive movements, or general stress. Regularly performing shoulder rolls can help in enhancing shoulder flexibility, reducing tension, and improving posture.

Instructions for Shoulder Rolls

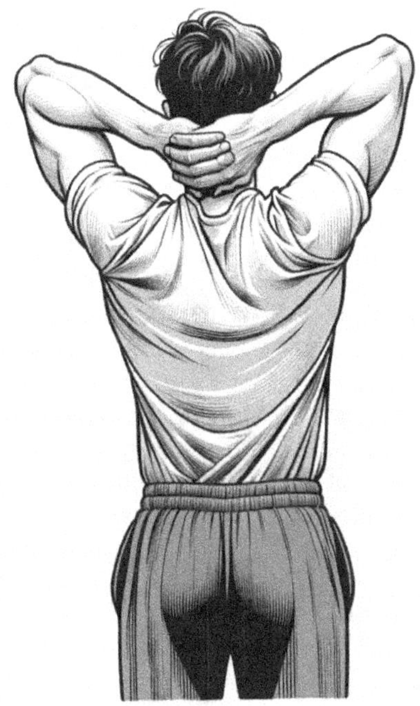

1. Starting Position:

   - Stand or sit upright with your feet flat on the floor.

   - Keep your arms relaxed at your sides.

2. Performing the Exercise:

   - Slowly lift your shoulders up towards your ears.

   - Gently roll your shoulders back, squeezing your shoulder blades together.

- Continue the motion by bringing your shoulders down and then forward, completing the circle.
- Ensure the movements are smooth and controlled.

3. Breathing:
-Take a breath and raise your shoulders.
- Let out a breath when you raise and lower your shoulders.

Number of Sets and Repetitions
- • - Repeat the shoulder rolls for 8-10 repetitions.
- • - Perform 2-3 sets.

Frequency
- You can do this exercise daily, especially if you spend long periods in a seated position or engage in activities that strain the shoulders.

Remember to maintain a relaxed posture throughout the exercise, avoiding any strain or discomfort. Regular practice of shoulder rolls can greatly contribute to shoulder health and overall well-being.

Here is an illustration showing a person performing the Arm Raises exercise. Now, let's discuss the details of this exercise.

Arm Raises

Arm Raises are a simple yet effective exercise for strengthening the shoulder muscles and improving upper body mobility. In my experience as a gym instructor, I've found Arm Raises to be particularly beneficial for people who want to improve their upper body strength and posture, as well as for those who engage in activities that require good shoulder mobility.

Instructions for Arm Raises

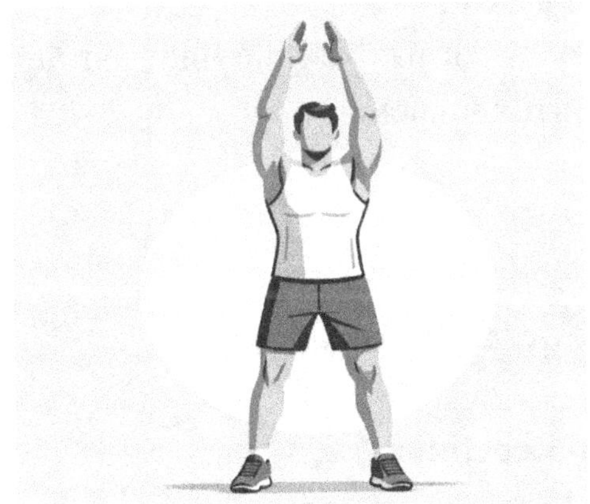

1. Starting Position:
   - Stand with your feet shoulder-width apart, or sit upright in a chair.
   - Keep your arms at your sides, palms facing inwards.

2. Performing the Exercise:
   - Slowly lift your arms straight up in front of you, keeping them parallel to each other.
   - Continue raising your arms until they are level with your head or as high as comfortable.
   - Maintain a straight arm position without locking your elbows. - At the peak of the movement, pause momentarily.

3. Lowering the Arms:
   - Slowly lower your arms back to the starting position in a controlled manner.

4. Breathing:
   - Inhale as you lift your arms up.
   - Exhale as you lower them back down.

Number of Sets and Repetitions
   - - Perform 8-12 repetitions of the exercise.

- - Aim for 2-3 sets.

Frequency
- This exercise can be done 2-3 times a week as part of an upper body workout routine.

It's important to keep your movements controlled and avoid any jerky motions. If you're new to this exercise or have shoulder issues, start with a smaller range of motion and gradually increase it as you become more comfortable. Regular practice of Arm Raises can help in building shoulder strength and enhancing overall upper body fitness.

Gentle Spinal Twists

Gentle Spinal Twists are an excellent exercise for increasing spinal mobility and relieving tension in the back. As a gym instructor, I often recommend this exercise to individuals seeking to improve their spinal health, particularly those who spend long periods sitting. This exercise can help in loosening the muscles around the spine, promoting better posture and reducing back discomfort.

Instructions for Gentle Spinal Twists

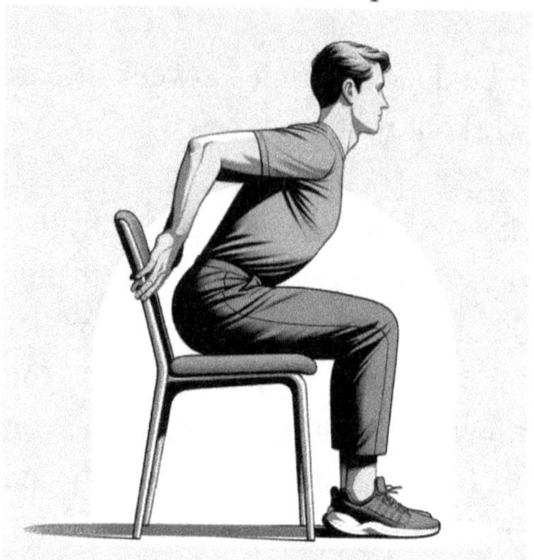

1. Starting Position:

  - Sit upright in a chair, feet flat on the floor, and spine elongated.

  - Keep your hands resting on your thighs.

2. Performing the Exercise:

  - Place your left hand on your right knee.

  - Bring your right hand to the back of the chair for support or both hands if comfortable.

  - Gently twist your torso to the right, starting from the base of your spine.

  - Turn your head to look over your right shoulder if it's comfortable.

- Keep the twist gentle and avoid straining.

3. Holding the Pose:
 - Hold the twist for 15-30 seconds, breathing deeply and evenly.

4. Returning to Center and Repeating:
 - Slowly come back to the center.
 - Repeat the twist on the opposite side, placing your right hand on your left knee and twisting to the left.

Number of Sets and Repetitions
- - Perform the twist 2-3 times on each side.
- - You can do this exercise 1-2 times a day, especially if you experience back stiffness.

It's important to keep the movements gentle and controlled. The focus should be on feeling a comfortable stretch along the spine rather than pushing into a deep twist. Regular practice of Gentle Spinal Twists can greatly contribute to spinal health and overall well-being.

Ankle Circles

Ankle Circles are a straightforward yet highly effective exercise for improving ankle mobility and circulation. In my experience as a gym instructor, I've seen how beneficial this exercise can be, especially for those who spend a lot of time seated or have limited mobility. Regularly performing ankle circles can help in reducing stiffness, preventing ankle injuries, and improving overall foot health.

Instructions for Ankle Circles

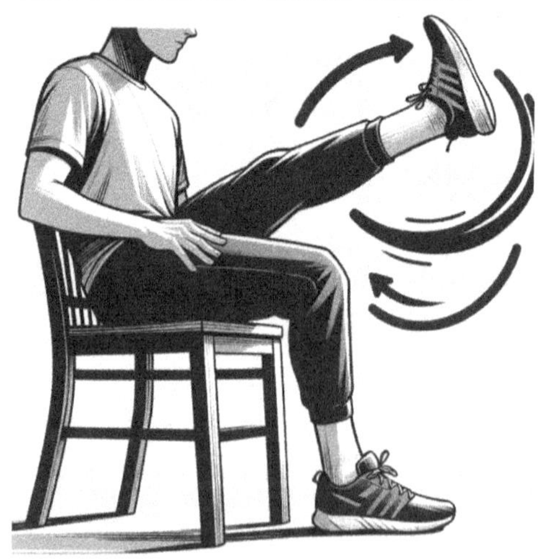

1. Starting Position:

- Sit comfortably in a chair with your feet flat on the floor.
- Straighten one leg out in front of you, keeping the other foot on the floor for balance.

2. Performing the Exercise:
- Lift your extended leg slightly off the ground or go higher if comfortable.
- Begin rotating your ankle slowly in a circular motion.
- Focus on making smooth, controlled circles with your ankle.

3. Direction and Repetitions:
- Rotate your ankle 10 times in one direction.
- Then switch and rotate 10 times in the opposite direction.
- Lower your leg back to the starting position.

4. Repeat with the Other Ankle:
- Repeat the same process with your other ankle.

Number of Sets and Repetitions
- Perform 2-3 sets on each ankle.

Frequency

- You can do this exercise daily, especially if you experience stiffness or swelling in the ankles.

Ankle Circles are particularly useful for improving joint mobility and can be easily incorporated into your daily routine. They are an excellent exercise for people of all ages and fitness levels, providing a gentle way to keep the ankles strong and flexible.

Seated Cat-Cow Stretch

The Seated Cat-Cow Stretch is a gentle, effective exercise for enhancing spinal flexibility and relieving tension in the back and neck. Adapted from traditional yoga, this seated version is perfect for those who spend long hours sitting or have limited mobility. As a gym instructor, I've found that this exercise is excellent for improving posture and encouraging a greater range of motion in the spine.

Instructions for Seated Cat-Cow Stretch

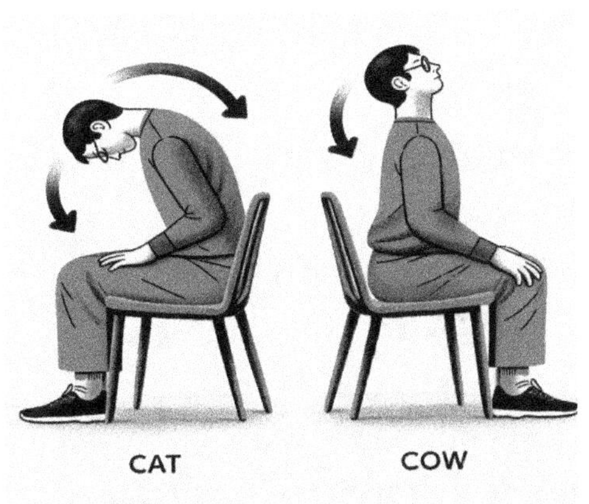

1. Starting Position:

  - Sit upright in a chair with your feet flat on the floor.

  - Place your hands on your knees or thighs.

2. Cat Phase:

  - Exhale and gently arch your spine upwards.

  - Tuck your chin towards your chest, rounding your shoulders forward.

  - Feel the stretch along your back.

3. Cow Phase:

  - Inhale and curve your spine downwards.

  - Lift your chin and chest upwards, pulling your shoulders back.

  - This position should create a gentle stretch in your chest and neck.

4. Flowing Between Phases:
  - Alternate between the Cat and Cow phases, moving with your breath.
  - Exhale as you move into the Cat stretch, and inhale into the Cow stretch.

Number of Sets and Repetitions
- - Perform the stretch for 8-10 repetitions.
- - Aim for 2-3 sets.

Frequency
- This exercise can be done daily, especially as a break from prolonged sitting.

The Seated Cat-Cow Stretch is not only beneficial for the spine but also helps in calming the mind and reducing stress. Remember to move gently, allowing your breath to guide the movement, and avoid pushing into any pain or discomfort. Regular practice can contribute significantly to spinal health and overall well-being.

Forward Bend and Reach

The Forward Bend and Reach is a gentle exercise that helps in stretching the back, shoulders, and hamstrings. Particularly beneficial for those who sit for extended periods, this exercise aids in relieving tension in the lower back and improving overall flexibility. As a gym instructor, I recommend this exercise for its effectiveness in enhancing spinal mobility and reducing stiffness.

Instructions for Forward Bend and Reach

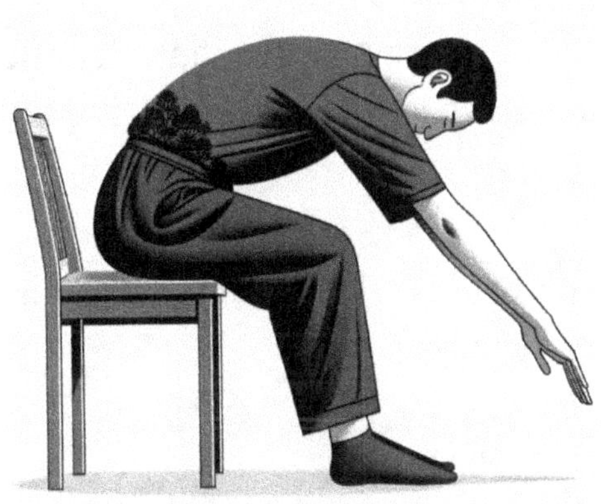

1. Starting Position:

- Place your feet hip-width apart and flat on the floor while seated in a chair. With your hands resting on your thighs, adopt a straight posture.

2. Performing the Exercise:
   - Inhale deeply, and as you exhale, slowly bend forward from your hips.
   - Extend your arms straight ahead, reaching towards your feet.
   - Keep your back as straight as possible, and look downwards towards your knees.
   - Reach as far as comfortable, feeling a gentle stretch in your back and legs.

3. Holding the Pose:
   - Hold the forward bend for a few seconds, continuing to breathe deeply.

4. Returning to Starting Position:
   - Slowly come back up to the sitting position as you inhale.

Number of Sets and Repetitions
   - - Perform this stretch for 8-10 repetitions.
   - - Aim for 2-3 sets.

Frequency
- This exercise can be performed daily, especially if you experience lower back tightness or stiffness.

The Forward Bend and Reach is a simple yet effective exercise that can be easily incorporated into your daily routine. It's important to move into and out of the stretch slowly and with control, avoiding any jerky movements. Regular practice can help maintain spinal health, improve posture, and enhance overall well-being.

CHAPTER 4: UPPER BODY EXERCISES

Seated Shoulder Press

The Seated Shoulder Press is a strength-building exercise targeting the shoulders and upper arms. This exercise is particularly effective for improving upper body strength and enhancing muscle tone. Performing this exercise while seated helps maintain good posture and provides stability, making it suitable for a wide range of fitness levels.

Instructions for Seated Shoulder Press

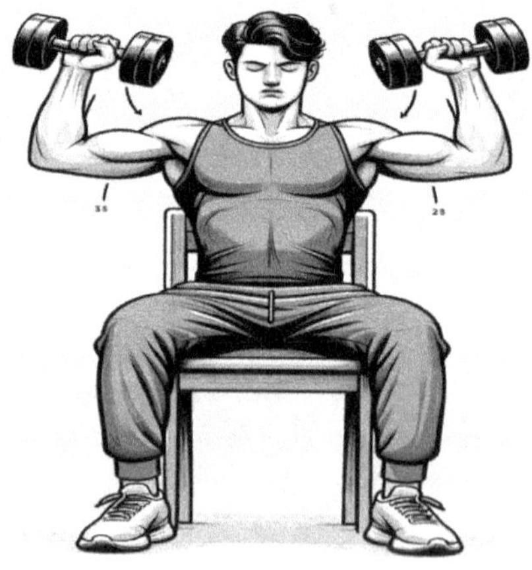

1. Starting Position:
   - Sit in a chair with your back straight and feet flat on the floor.
   - Hold a weight in each hand at shoulder height, with elbows bent and palms facing forward.

2. Performing the Exercise:
   - Exhale and press the weights upwards until your arms are fully extended above your head.
   - Keep your wrists straight and avoid locking your elbows at the top of the movement.
   - Pause briefly at the top.

3. Lowering the Weights:
   - Inhale and slowly lower the weights back to shoulder height.

Number of Sets and Repetitions
   - - Perform 8-12 repetitions per set.
   - - Aim for 2-3 sets of this exercise.

Frequency
- Include this exercise in your upper body workouts, ideally 2-3 times a week.

It's important to choose a weight that challenges your muscles while still allowing you to maintain good form.If you've never done this kind of exercise before, begin with less weights and work your way up as your strength increases. Regular practice of the Seated Shoulder Press can lead to significant improvements in shoulder strength and overall upper body conditioning.

Chair Push-Ups

Chair Push-Ups are a modified version of the classic push-up, performed using a chair to reduce the intensity. This exercise is excellent for strengthening the chest, shoulders, and triceps while being more accessible than floor push-ups. It's particularly beneficial for those building upper body strength or for individuals who find traditional push-ups too challenging.

Instructions for Chair Push-Ups

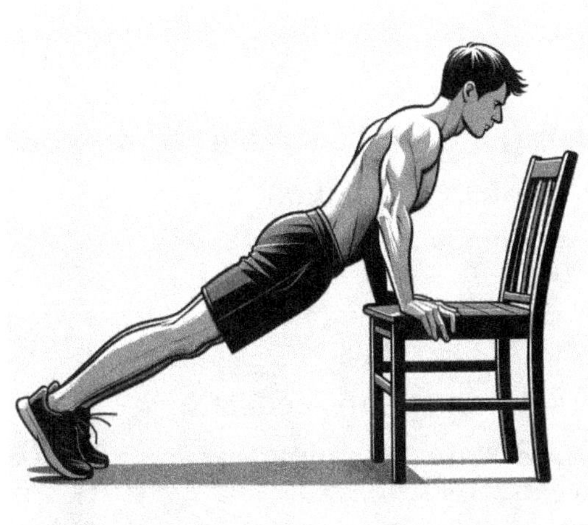

1. Starting Position:

   - Place a sturdy chair against a wall for stability.

   - Stand facing the chair and place your hands on the edge of the seat, slightly wider than shoulder-width apart.

   - Step your feet back until your body forms a straight line from your head to your heels, similar to a plank position.

2. Performing the Exercise:

   - Inhale and bend your elbows to lower your chest towards the chair.

   - Keep your body straight and core engaged.

- Lower down until your chest is close to the chair, but without touching it.

3. Pushing Up:
   - Exhale and push through your hands to lift your body back up to the starting position.
   - Keep your movements controlled.

Number of Sets and Repetitions
  - - Perform 8-15 repetitions per set.
  - - Aim for 2-3 sets, depending on your fitness level.

Frequency
- Include this exercise in your upper body routine 2-3 times a week.

It's important to choose a chair that is stable and can support your weight. As you gain strength, you can increase the number of repetitions or sets, or progress to more challenging variations. Chair Push-Ups are an effective way to build upper body strength and improve muscular endurance.

Bicep Curls

Bicep Curls are a popular strength training exercise focused on building the biceps muscles in the upper arms. This exercise is effective for increasing arm strength and improving muscular definition. Performing Bicep Curls while seated helps maintain good posture and focuses the effort on the biceps without involving the back muscles.

Instructions for Bicep Curls

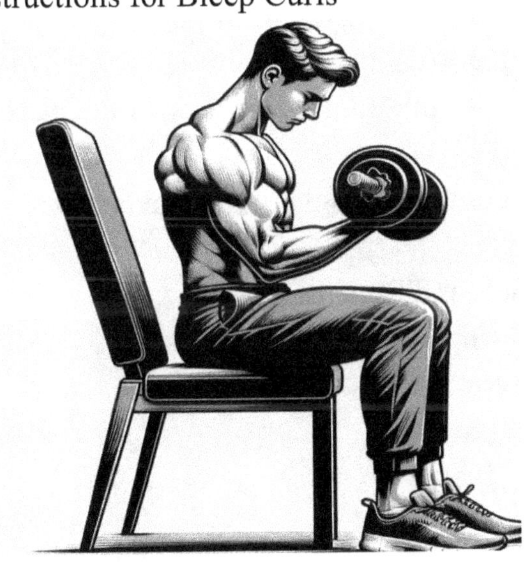

1. Starting Position:
   - Sit in a chair with your feet flat on the floor and your back straight.
   - Hold a dumbbell in each hand with your arms down at your sides, palms facing forward.

2. Performing the Curl:
   - Keep your upper arms stationary, and bend your elbows to curl the weights up towards your shoulders.
   - Contract your biceps as you lift the weights.
   - Ensure that only your forearms are moving.

3. Lowering the Weights:
   - Slowly lower the dumbbells back to the starting position.
   - Maintain control throughout the movement.

Number of Sets and Repetitions
   - - Perform 8-12 repetitions per set.
   - - Aim for 2-3 sets.

Frequency

- Include this exercise in your arm or upper body strength routine, typically 2-3 times a week.

It's important to select a weight that allows you to complete each set with good form. If the weight is too heavy, it can lead to compensating with other muscles or swinging the weights, which reduces the effectiveness of the exercise. Regular practice of Bicep Curls can significantly enhance arm strength and muscle tone.

Tricep Dips

Tricep Dips are an effective bodyweight exercise that targets the triceps muscles in the upper arms. This exercise is excellent for strengthening and toning the arms, particularly the triceps. Performing Tricep Dips using a chair is a convenient way to do this exercise almost anywhere, making it a popular choice for home workouts.

Instructions for Tricep Dips

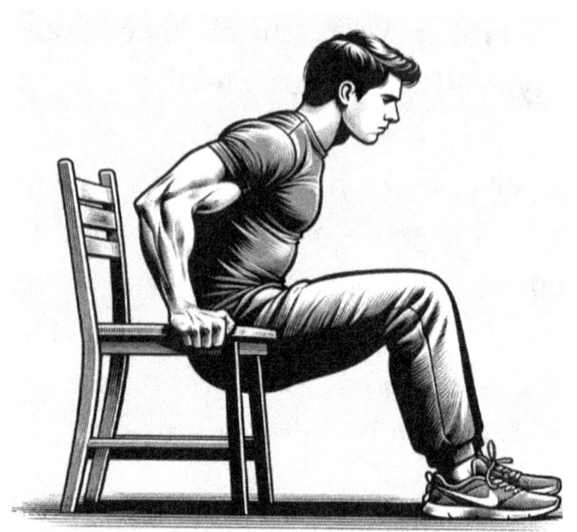

1. Starting Position:

   - Sit on the edge of a sturdy chair with your hands gripping the front edge beside your hips.

   - Extend your legs forward, feet flat on the floor, and knees bent so that your legs are perpendicular to the floor.

2. Performing the Dip:

   - Slide your hips off the chair, supporting your weight with your arms.

   - Lower your body by bending your elbows to about a 90-degree angle, keeping your back close to the chair.

   - Your shoulders should be down and away from your ears.

3. Rising Up:
   - To straighten your arms and raise your body back to the beginning position, push through your hands.

Number of Sets and Repetitions
- Aim for 8-12 repetitions per set.
- Perform 2-3 sets, depending on your fitness level.

Frequency
- You can include Tricep Dips in your upper body workout routine, 2-3 times a week.

It's important to keep the movement controlled and to avoid locking your elbows when you come to the top of the dip. Start with fewer repetitions and sets if you're new to this exercise and gradually increase as your strength improves. Regular practice of Tricep Dips can lead to significant improvements in upper arm strength and muscle definition.

Seated Chest Fly

The Seated Chest Fly is an effective exercise for strengthening and toning the chest muscles (pectoralis major and minor). This is a great exercise to strengthen your upper body and correct your posture. Performing this exercise while seated helps in maintaining good spinal alignment and focuses the effort on the chest muscles.

Instructions for Seated Chest Fly

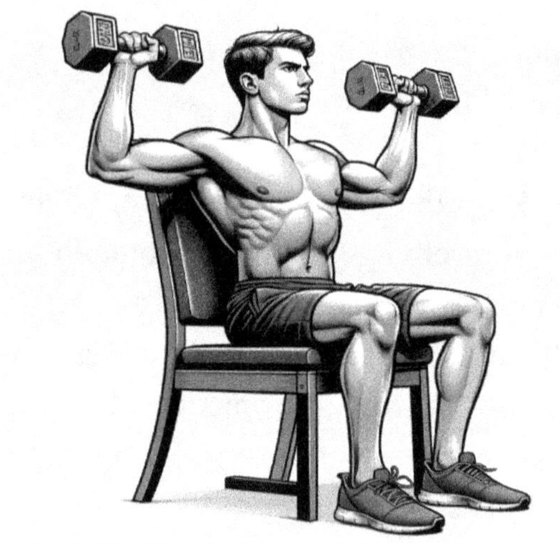

1. Starting Position:
   - Sit in a chair with your back straight and feet flat on the floor.

- Hold a dumbbell in each hand, arms extended out to the sides at shoulder height, with elbows slightly bent.

2. Performing the Exercise:
- Slowly bring the dumbbells together in front of your chest. Keep your arms at shoulder height and elbows slightly bent throughout the movement.
- Squeeze your chest muscles as the dumbbells come together.
- Pause briefly when your hands are in front of your chest.

3. Returning to Starting Position:
- Slowly open your arms back to the starting position in a controlled manner.

Number of Sets and Repetitions
- Beginners: Aim for 6-8 repetitions per set, 1-2 sets.
- Intermediate: Perform 8-12 repetitions per set, 2-3 sets.
- Advanced: Aim for 12-15 repetitions per set, 3-4 sets.

Frequency
- Include this exercise in your upper body workout routine, ideally 2-3 times a week.

Choose a weight that allows you to complete each set with good form. If the weight is too heavy, it can compromise your form and reduce the effectiveness of the exercise. Regular practice of the Seated Chest Fly can lead to significant improvements in chest strength and muscle tone.

Front Arm Raises

Front Arm Raises are an effective exercise for strengthening the shoulder muscles, particularly the anterior deltoids. This exercise is beneficial for improving upper body strength and shoulder stability. Performing this exercise while seated helps maintain proper posture and focuses the effort on the shoulder muscles.

Instructions for Front Arm Raises

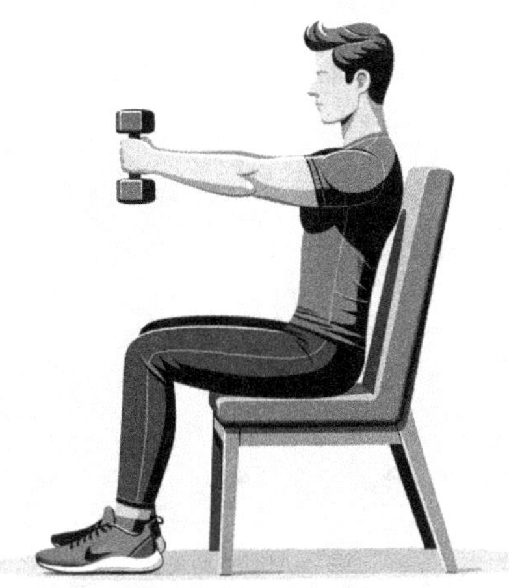

1. Starting Position:

- Sit in a chair with your back straight and feet flat on the floor.

- Hold a dumbbell in each hand, arms extended down at your sides, palms facing your thighs.

2. Performing the Exercise:

- Slowly lift the weights straight up in front of you, keeping your arms straight.

- Raise the dumbbells to shoulder height, ensuring not to lift them too high.

- Keep your back straight and avoid leaning backward.

3. Lowering the Weights:
   - Slowly lower the dumbbells back to the starting position in a controlled manner.

Number of Sets and Repetitions
- - Beginners: Aim for 6-8 repetitions per set, 1-2 sets.
- - Intermediate: Perform 8-12 repetitions per set, 2-3 sets.
- - Advanced: Aim for 12-15 repetitions per set, 3-4 sets.

Frequency
- Include this exercise in your shoulder or upper body workout routine, ideally 2-3 times a week.

Select a weight that allows you to complete each set with good form. If the weight is too heavy, it can lead to compensating with other muscles, reducing the effectiveness of the exercise. Regular practice of Front Arm Raises can significantly enhance shoulder strength and muscle definition.

Lateral Arm Raises

Lateral Arm Raises are a targeted exercise for strengthening the shoulder muscles, specifically the lateral deltoids. This exercise is important for building shoulder strength and stability, and enhancing the overall shape of the shoulders. Performing Lateral Arm Raises while seated helps in maintaining proper posture and isolates the shoulder muscles effectively.

Instructions for Lateral Arm Raises

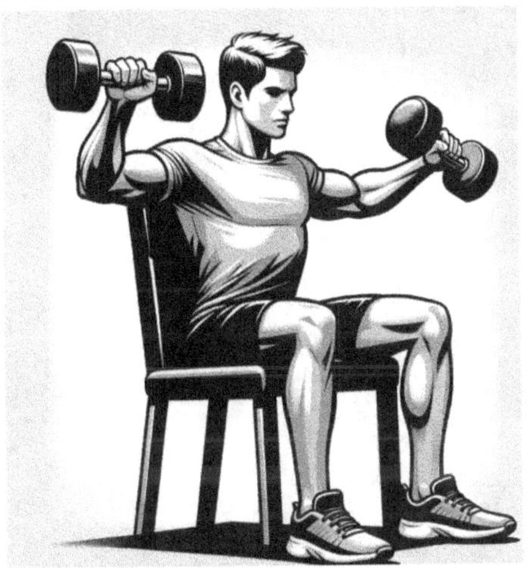

1. Starting Position:
   - Sit in a chair with your back straight and feet flat on the floor.

- Hold a dumbbell in each hand, arms extended down at your sides, palms facing inward.

2. Performing the Exercise:
  - Lift the weights out to the sides, keeping your arms straight.
  - Raise the dumbbells to shoulder height, ensuring not to lift them too high.
  - Your palms should be facing down at the top of the movement.

3. Lowering the Weights:
  - Slowly lower the dumbbells back to the starting position in a controlled manner.

Number of Sets and Repetitions
  - - Beginners: Aim for 6-8 repetitions per set, 1-2 sets.
  - - Intermediate: Perform 8-12 repetitions per set, 2-3 sets.
  - - Advanced: Aim for 12-15 repetitions per set, 3-4 sets.

Frequency
- Include this exercise in your shoulder or upper body workout routine, ideally 2-3 times a week.

Choosing the right weight is crucial. It should be heavy enough to challenge your muscles but light enough to allow for proper form throughout the exercise. Regular practice of Lateral Arm Raises can lead to significant improvements in shoulder strength and muscular definition.

Seated Rows

Seated Rows are a great exercise for strengthening the back muscles, particularly the middle and upper back. This exercise also engages the biceps and helps in improving posture. Using a resistance band for Seated Rows while seated in a chair is a convenient and effective way to perform this exercise, making it suitable for a variety of fitness levels.

Instructions for Seated Rows

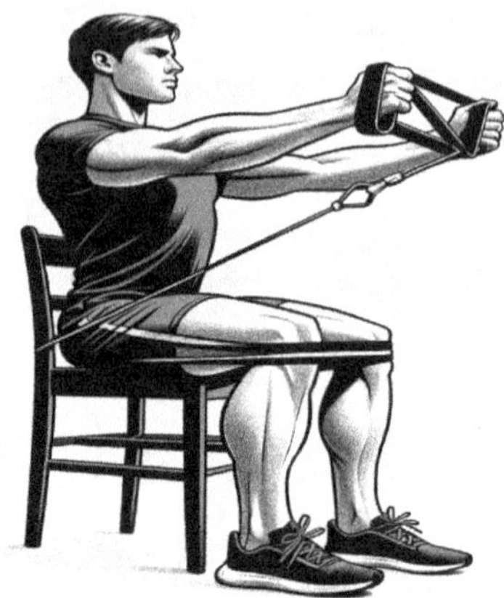

1. Starting Position:

   - Sit on a chair with your back straight and feet flat on the floor.

   - Loop a resistance band around your feet and hold each end with your hands.

2. Performing the Exercise:

   - With your arms extended, pull the band towards your waist.

   - Keep your elbows bent and close to your body.

   - Squeeze your shoulder blades together as you pull the band.

3. Returning to Starting Position:

- Slowly extend your arms back to the starting position, maintaining control.

Number of Sets and Repetitions
- *Beginners: Aim for 8-10 repetitions per set, 1-2 sets.*
- *Intermediate: Perform 10-12 repetitions per set, 2-3 sets.*
- *Advanced: Aim for 12-15 repetitions per set, 3-4 sets.*

Frequency
- Include Seated Rows in your upper body or back workout routine, ideally 2-3 times a week.

It's important to select a resistance band with the appropriate level of tension. The band should provide resistance but allow you to complete each set with good form. Regular practice of Seated Rows can significantly enhance back strength and improve upper body posture.

Reverse Flys

Reverse Flys are an effective exercise for targeting the muscles of the upper back, particularly the rear deltoids and the rhomboids. This exercise is beneficial for improving posture, shoulder stability, and overall upper body strength. Performing Reverse Flys while seated ensures proper alignment and focuses the effort on the targeted muscles.

Instructions for Reverse Flys

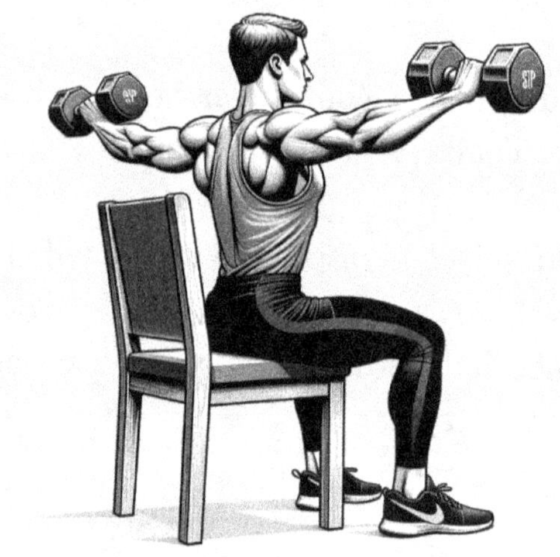

1. Starting Position:
   - Sit on the edge of a chair with your feet flat on the floor.
   - Lean forward slightly from the waist with a straight back.

- Hold a dumbbell in each hand, arms extended down and palms facing each other.

2. Performing the Exercise:
- Lift the weights out to the sides, keeping your arms slightly bent.
- Raise the dumbbells to shoulder height, but not higher, to maintain focus on the upper back muscles.
- Your shoulder blades should move towards each other as you lift the weights.

3. Returning to Starting Position:
- Slowly lower the dumbbells back to the starting position in a controlled manner.

Number of Sets and Repetitions
- - Beginners: Aim for 6-8 repetitions per set, 1-2 sets.
- - Intermediate: Perform 8-12 repetitions per set, 2-3 sets.
- - Advanced: Aim for 12-15 repetitions per set, 3-4 sets.

Frequency
- Include Reverse Flys in your upper body or back workout routine, ideally 2-3 times a week.

Choose weights that allow you to complete each set with proper form. The exercise should be challenging but not compromise your posture or control. Regular practice of Reverse Flys can significantly enhance upper back strength and contribute to a well-balanced and toned upper body.

Upright Rows

Upright Rows are a strength training exercise that primarily targets the shoulders, specifically the traps and deltoids, as well as the upper back. This exercise is effective for enhancing shoulder strength and improving upper body muscle definition. Performing Upright Rows while seated helps in maintaining good posture and isolates the shoulder muscles more effectively.

Instructions for Upright Rows

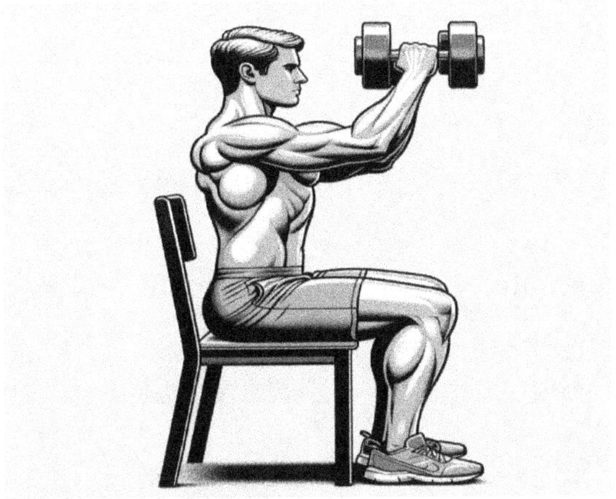

1. Starting Position:

   - Sit in a chair with your back straight and feet flat on the floor.

   - Hold a dumbbell in each hand in front of you, arms extended downwards, palms facing your body.

2. Performing the Exercise:

   - Lift the weights straight up along your body towards your chin.

   - Keep your elbows leading the movement and pointing outwards.

   - Lift the dumbbells to just below chin height, ensuring your elbows are higher than your forearms.

3. Lowering the Weights:

- Slowly lower the dumbbells back to the starting position in a controlled manner.

Number of Sets and Repetitions
- • - Beginners: Aim for 6-8 repetitions per set, 1-2 sets.
- • - Intermediate: Perform 8-12 repetitions per set, 2-3 sets.
- • - Advanced: Aim for 12-15 repetitions per set, 3-4 sets.

Frequency
- Include Upright Rows in your upper body workout routine, ideally 2-3 times a week.

Select weights that are challenging but allow you to maintain good form throughout the exercise. Avoid lifting the dumbbells too high, which can strain the shoulders. Regular practice of Upright Rows can significantly improve shoulder strength and contribute to a well-toned upper body.

CHAPTER 5: LOWER BODY EXERCISES

Seated Leg Lifts

Seated Leg Lifts are a simple yet effective exercise for strengthening the thigh and hip flexor muscles. This exercise is particularly beneficial for improving leg strength and mobility. Performing Seated Leg Lifts is also great for those who spend a lot of time sitting, as it helps in activating the muscles that may be underused due to prolonged sitting.

Instructions for Seated Leg Lifts

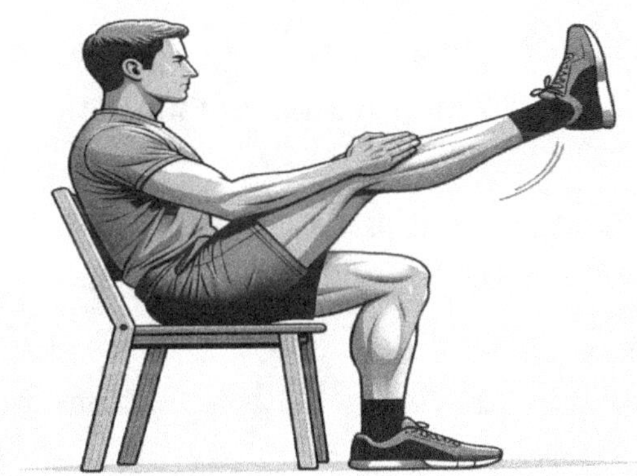

1. Starting Position:

- Sit in a chair with your back straight and feet flat on the floor.

- Place your hands on the sides of the chair for stability.

2. Performing the Exercise:

- Lift one leg straight out in front of you, keeping the knee straight and toe pointed.

- Raise the leg as high as you can while keeping your upper body still and stable.

- Hold the lifted position for a moment.

3. Lowering the Leg:

- Return your leg to the beginning position slowly and deliberately.

4. Repeating with the Other Leg:

- Perform the same motion with the other leg.

Number of Sets and Repetitions

- - Beginners: Aim for 6-8 repetitions per leg, 1-2 sets.

- - Intermediate: Perform 8-12 repetitions per leg, 2-3 sets.

- - Advanced: Aim for 12-15 repetitions per leg, 3-4 sets.

Frequency
- Include Seated Leg Lifts in your lower body or general fitness routine, ideally 2-3 times a week.

It's important to keep your movements controlled and to focus on using your thigh muscles to lift your leg. This exercise can be performed without weights for beginners and weights can be added for increased difficulty as you progress. Regular practice of Seated Leg Lifts can significantly improve leg strength and contribute to overall lower body fitness.

Chair Squats

Chair Squats are an excellent exercise for strengthening the lower body, particularly the quadriceps, hamstrings, and glutes. This exercise is a modified version of the traditional squat, using a chair as a guide to ensure proper form and depth. It's ideal for those new to squats or anyone looking to add a safe and effective lower body exercise to their routine.

Instructions for Chair Squats

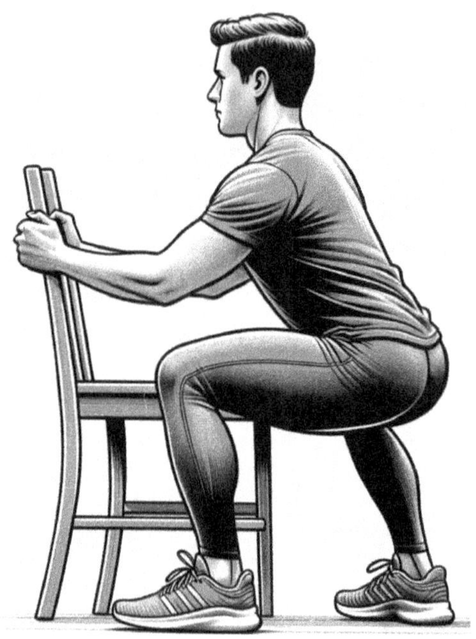

1. Starting Position:

   - Stand in front of a chair with your feet shoulder-width apart, facing the chair.

   - Keep your back straight, chest up, and arms extended forward for balance using the chair for support.

2. Performing the Exercise:

- Begin by slowly bending your knees and pushing your hips back as if you are going to sit down.

- Lower your body towards the chair, stopping just above the seat.

- Ensure your knees do not go past your toes and your weight is on your heels.

3. Rising Up:

- Push through your heels to lift your body back up to the starting position.

Number of Sets and Repetitions

- - Beginners: Aim for 8-10 repetitions per set, 1-2 sets.
- - Intermediate: Perform 10-12 repetitions per set, 2-3 sets.
- - Advanced: Aim for 12-15 repetitions per set, 3-4 sets.

Frequency
- Include Chair Squats in your lower body workout routine, ideally 2-3 times a week.

It's important to perform this exercise with control, focusing on maintaining proper form to maximize its benefits and minimize the risk of injury. Chair

Squats are a versatile exercise that can be adjusted in intensity by adding weights or increasing the speed of the movements. Regular practice can lead to significant improvements in lower body strength and muscle tone.

Seated Knee Raises

Seated Knee Raises are a gentle yet effective exercise primarily targeting the core and hip flexor muscles. This exercise is especially beneficial for those who may have difficulty standing or performing high-impact activities. It's a great way to engage and strengthen the abdominal muscles and improve lower body mobility while seated.

Instructions for Seated Knee Raises

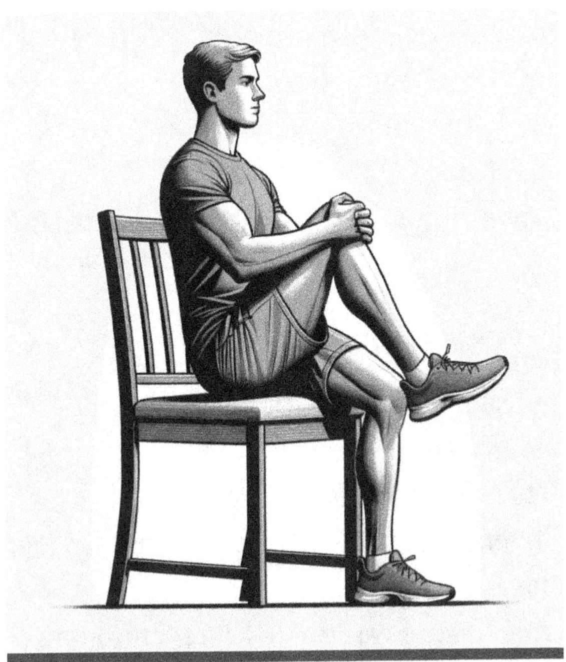

1. Starting Position:

   - Sit in a chair with your back straight and feet flat on the floor.

   - Place your hands on the sides of the chair for support.

2. Performing the Exercise:

   - Lift one knee towards your chest as high as comfortably as possible.

   - You may hold your knee with both hands for a brief moment to deepen the engagement of the core muscles.

- Keep the movement controlled and focus on using your abdominal muscles to lift your knee.

3. Lowering the Knee:
- Gently lower your leg back to the starting position.

4. Repeating with the Other Leg:
- Perform the same motion with the other leg.

Number of Sets and Repetitions
- - Beginners: Aim for 6-8 repetitions per leg, 1-2 sets.
- - Intermediate: Perform 8-12 repetitions per leg, 2-3 sets.
- - Advanced: Aim for 12-15 repetitions per leg, 3-4 sets.

Frequency
- Include Seated Knee Raises in your core or lower body routine, ideally 2-3 times a week.

This exercise can be adapted to various fitness levels by adjusting the number of repetitions and sets. Regular practice of Seated Knee Raises can lead to improved core strength and better stability, which is essential for overall mobility and balance.

Ankle Weights Leg Extension

Ankle Weights Leg Extension is a strength-building exercise targeting the quadriceps muscles in the front of the thigh. The addition of ankle weights increases resistance, enhancing muscle engagement and strength development. This exercise is excellent for improving leg strength and muscle tone, and can be particularly beneficial for those who spend a lot of time seated.

Instructions for Ankle Weights Leg Extension

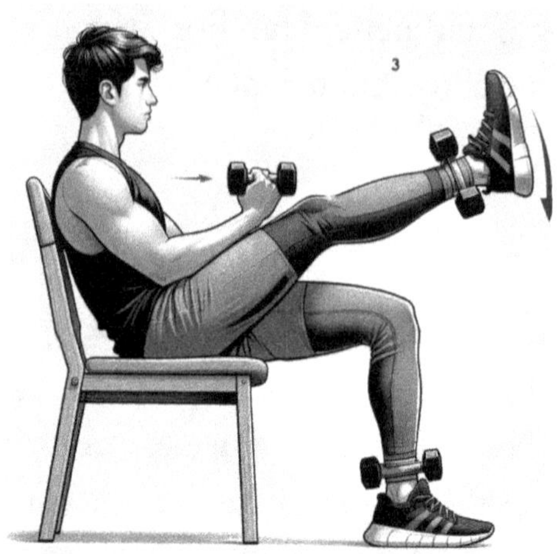

1. Starting Position:

   - Sit in a chair with your back straight and feet flat on the floor.

   - Secure ankle weights around both ankles.

2. Performing the Exercise:

   - Lift one leg and extend it straight out in front of you, keeping your knee straight.

   - Extend your leg as far as you can, focusing on contracting the quadriceps.

   - Keep the movement controlled and smooth.

3. Returning to Starting Position:

   - Slowly lower your leg back to the starting position.

4. Repeating with the Other Leg:
   - Perform the same motion with the other leg.

Number of Sets and Repetitions
- - Beginners: Aim for 6-8 repetitions per leg, 1-2 sets.
- - Intermediate: Perform 8-12 repetitions per leg, 2-3 sets.
- - Advanced: Aim for 12-15 repetitions per leg, 3-4 sets.

Frequency
- Include this exercise in your lower body or overall fitness routine, ideally 2-3 times a week.

The use of ankle weights adds resistance, making the exercise more challenging. It's important to start with a weight that is manageable and gradually increase as your strength improves. Regular practice of Ankle Weights Leg Extension can significantly enhance leg strength, muscle tone, and overall lower body fitness.

Calf Raises

Calf Raises are a fundamental exercise for strengthening the calf muscles (gastrocnemius and soleus). This exercise is key for improving lower leg strength, ankle stability, and balance. It can be particularly beneficial for activities that involve running or walking, as well as for overall leg toning.

Instructions for Calf Raises

1. Starting Position:
   - Stand behind a chair and use it for support, keeping your feet flat on the floor.
   - Place your feet hip-width apart.

2. Performing the Exercise:
   - Slowly raise your heels off the floor, standing on your toes.
   - Engage your calf muscles as you rise to your tiptoes.
   - Keep your posture upright and focus on maintaining balance.

3. Lowering Back Down:
   - Gently lower your heels back to the floor.

Number of Sets and Repetitions
- • - Beginners: Aim for 8-10 repetitions, 1-2 sets.
- • - Intermediate: Perform 10-15 repetitions, 2-3 sets.
- • - Advanced: Aim for 15-20 repetitions, 3-4 sets.

Frequency
- You can perform Calf Raises 2-3 times a week as part of a lower body workout or general fitness routine.

Calf Raises are a simple yet effective exercise that can be easily incorporated into any fitness regimen. They require no special equipment and can be performed anywhere. Regular practice can lead to stronger calves, improved balance, and better performance in various physical activities.

Seated Hamstring Curls

Seated Hamstring Curls are an effective exercise for targeting and strengthening the hamstring muscles located at the back of the thigh. This exercise is particularly beneficial for individuals who may have difficulty standing or performing traditional hamstring exercises. It helps in improving leg strength, flexibility, and can aid in injury prevention.

Instructions for Seated Hamstring Curls

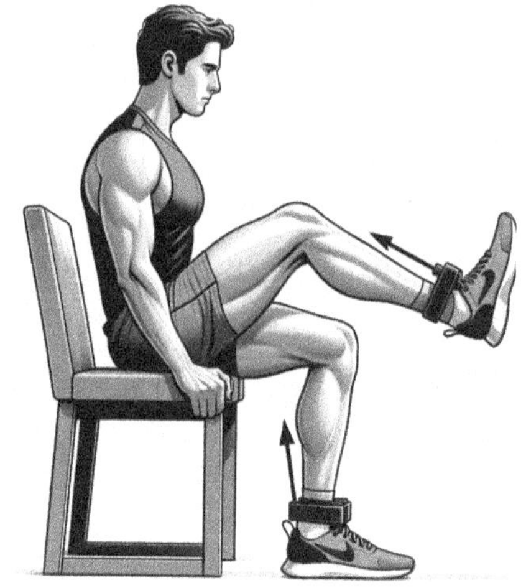

1. Starting Position:

   - Sit in a chair with your back straight and feet flat on the floor.

   - Secure ankle weights around both ankles.

2. Performing the Exercise:

- Lift one foot off the floor and bend your knee to curl your heel towards your buttocks.

- Focus on contracting the hamstring muscles as you perform the curl.

- Keep the movement controlled and avoid any jerky motions.

3. Returning to Starting Position:

- Slowly extend your leg back to the starting position.

4. Repeating with the Other Leg:

- Perform the same motion with the other leg.

Number of Sets and Repetitions

- - Beginners: Aim for 6-8 repetitions per leg, 1-2 sets.
- - Intermediate: Perform 8-12 repetitions per leg, 2-3 sets.
- - Advanced: Aim for 12-15 repetitions per leg, 3-4 sets.

Frequency

- Include Seated Hamstring Curls in your lower body or overall fitness routine, ideally 2-3 times a week.

The use of ankle weights adds resistance, making the exercise more challenging and effective. It's important to start with a manageable weight and gradually increase as your strength improves. Regular practice of Seated Hamstring Curls can significantly enhance hamstring strength and contribute to overall leg fitness.

Side Leg Raises

Side Leg Raises are a simple yet effective exercise targeting the muscles of the outer thigh and hips, known as the abductors. This exercise is excellent for improving hip stability, enhancing leg strength, and toning the outer thigh area. Performing Side Leg Raises while standing beside a chair provides balance and allows for a focused engagement of the target muscles.

Instructions for Side Leg Raises

1. Starting Position:
   - Stand beside a chair, using it for support.
   - Keep your feet close together and your posture upright.

2. Performing the Exercise:
   - Lift one leg out to the side, keeping the leg straight and toes pointed.
   - Raise your leg as high as comfortably possible without tilting your upper body.
   - Keep your supporting leg slightly bent for balance.

3. Returning to Starting Position:
   - Return your leg to the beginning position slowly and deliberately.

4. Repeating with the Other Leg:
   - Perform the same motion with the other leg.

Number of Sets and Repetitions
   - Beginners: Aim for 6-8 repetitions per leg, 1-2 sets.

- • - Intermediate: Perform 8-12 repetitions per leg, 2-3 sets.
- • - Advanced: Aim for 12-15 repetitions per leg, 3-4 sets.

Frequency
- Include Side Leg Raises in your lower body or overall fitness routine, ideally

Inner Thigh Squeezes
Inner Thigh Squeezes are a simple yet effective exercise targeting the adductor muscles, which are located in the inner thigh. This exercise is excellent for toning and strengthening these muscles, improving overall thigh strength, and enhancing stability. It's particularly beneficial as it can be performed while seated, making it accessible for a wide range of fitness levels.

Instructions for Inner Thigh Squeezes

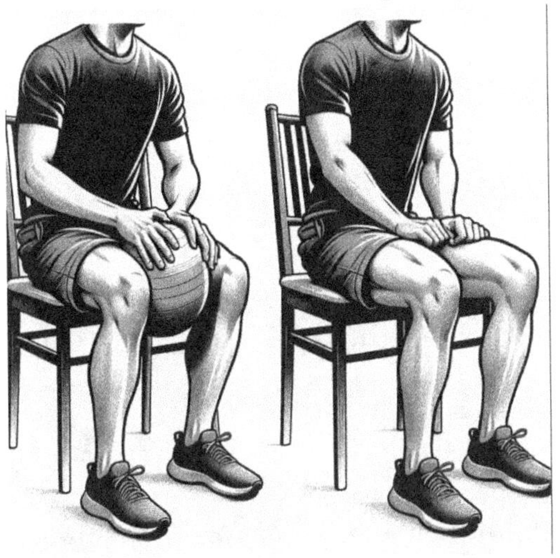

1. Starting Position:

   - Sit in a chair with your back straight and feet flat on the floor.

   - Place a small exercise ball or a folded towel between your knees.

2. Performing the Exercise:

   - Squeeze the ball or towel by pressing your knees together.

   - Focus on using your inner thigh muscles to apply the pressure.

   - Hold the squeeze for a few seconds.

3. Releasing the Squeeze:

- Slowly release the pressure and return to the starting position.

Number of Sets and Repetitions
- - Beginners: Aim for 8-10 squeezes, 1-2 sets.
- - Intermediate: Perform 10-15 squeezes, 2-3 sets.
- - Advanced: Aim for 15-20 squeezes, 3-4 sets.

Frequency
- Include Inner Thigh Squeezes in your lower body or general fitness routine, ideally 2-3 times a week.

This exercise can be easily incorporated into your daily routine, even while working at a desk or watching TV. Regular practice of Inner Thigh Squeezes can lead to stronger and more toned inner thigh muscles, contributing to better leg function and stability.

Toe Taps

Toe Taps are a simple, low-impact exercise that focuses on improving coordination and activating the muscles in the lower legs and feet. This exercise is especially beneficial for those looking to enhance foot dexterity, which is crucial for balance and mobility. Toe Taps can be easily performed while seated, making them a great addition to any low-intensity workout or as a gentle exercise for those with limited mobility.

Instructions for Toe Taps

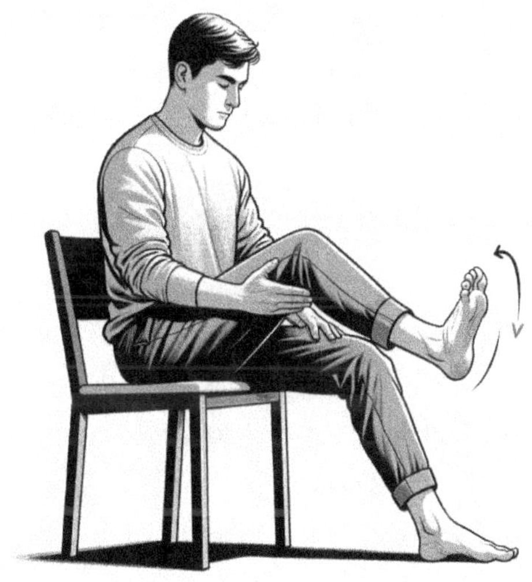

1. Starting Position:
   - Sit in a chair with your back straight and feet flat on the floor.
   - Keep your hands on your thighs or the sides of the chair for balance.

2. Performing the Exercise:
   - Lift one foot off the floor and tap your toe on the ground in front of you.
   - Lower your foot back to the starting position.
   - Alternate with the other foot, lifting and tapping in a steady, rhythmic motion.

3. Maintaining Posture:
   - Keep your upper body still and upright during the exercise.
   - Focus on the movement coming from your ankles and feet.

Number of Sets and Repetitions
- Beginners: Aim for 10-15 taps per foot, 1-2 sets.
- Intermediate: Perform 15-20 taps per foot, 2-3 sets.
- Advanced: Aim for 20-30 taps per foot, 3-4 sets.

Frequency
- Toe Taps can be done daily as a part of a routine to improve foot and ankle mobility.

This exercise is particularly useful for those who spend long periods sitting or have limited opportunity for physical activity. Regular practice of Toe Taps can lead to improved foot coordination, enhanced lower leg strength, and better overall mobility.

Seated Marching

Seated Marching is an accessible and beneficial exercise designed to engage the core and leg muscles, improving lower body mobility and coordination. It is particularly advantageous for individuals with limited standing ability or those seeking a low-impact exercise option. This exercise can be performed anywhere with a chair, making it a versatile addition to any fitness routine.

Instructions for Seated Marching

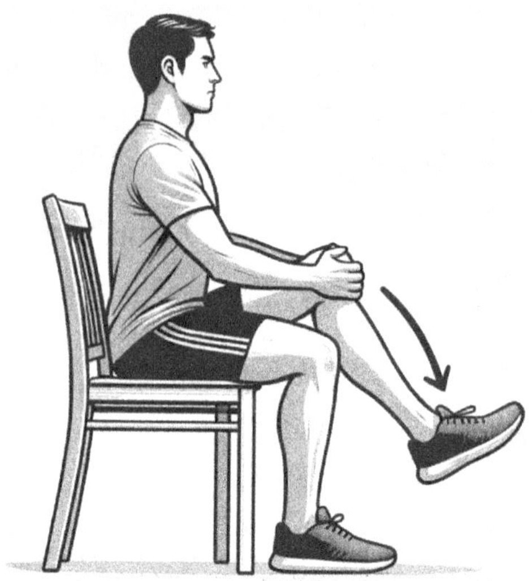

1. Starting Position:

- Sit in a chair with your back straight and feet flat on the floor.

- Place your hands on your thighs for stability.

2. Performing the Exercise:

- Lift one knee towards your chest, mimicking a marching motion.you may hold the lifted knee with your hands for support if comfortable.

- Lower the leg back to the floor and alternate with the other knee.

- Maintain an upright posture, engaging your core muscles as you lift each knee.

3. Breathing:
  - Inhale as you lift your knee and exhale as you lower it.

Number of Sets and Repetitions
- Beginners: Aim for 20-30 seconds per set, 1-2 sets.
- Intermediate: Perform 30-45 seconds per set, 2-3 sets.
- Advanced: Aim for 45-60 seconds per set, 3-4 sets.

Frequency
- Include Seated Marching in your daily routine or exercise regimen, ideally 2-3 times a week.

Seated Marching is excellent for stimulating circulation in the lower extremities and strengthening the muscles without placing undue stress on the joints. It is a simple yet effective way to maintain lower body strength and mobility, especially for those who spend long periods sitting. Regular practice can contribute to better leg function and overall physical health.

CHAPTER 6: FLEXIBILITY EXERCISES

Seated Spinal Twist

The Seated Spinal Twist is a rejuvenating stretch that targets the muscles of the spine, promoting flexibility and improving posture. This exercise is excellent for releasing tension in the back and can help in alleviating back discomfort. It's particularly beneficial for those who spend a lot of time sitting or who wish to enhance their core strength and spinal health.

Instructions for Seated Spinal Twist

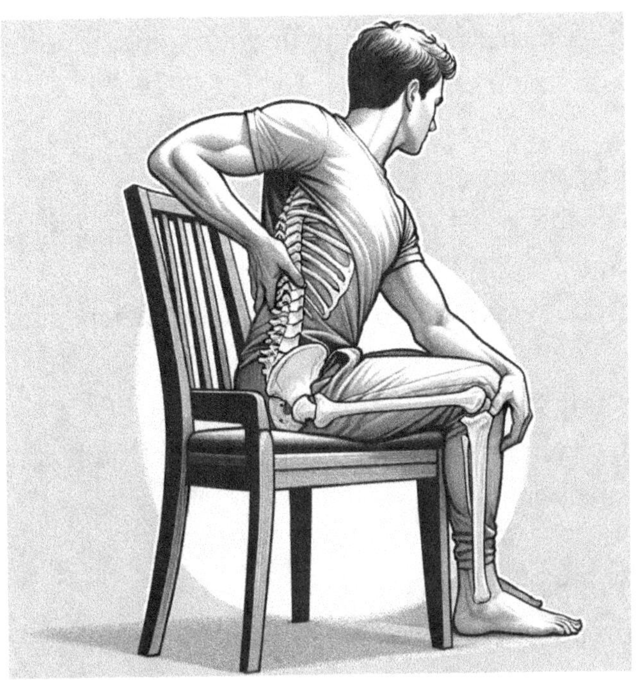

1. Starting Position:

   - Sit in a chair with your feet flat on the floor and your back straight.

   - Keep your hands resting on your thighs.

2. Performing the Twist:

   - Turn your torso to one side, placing one hand on the opposite knee and the other hand behind you or on the chair for support.

   - Ensure your twist initiates from the base of your spine, moving upwards through the vertebrae.

- Keep your head aligned with your spine, turning it in the direction of the twist.

3. Holding the Pose:
  - Hold the twist for 15-30 seconds, breathing deeply and steadily.
   - Focus on relaxing into the twist with each exhale.

4. Switching Sides:
  - Slowly return to the center and repeat the twist on the other side.

Number of Sets and Repetitions
- Perform the stretch once on each side.

Frequency
- Include the Seated Spinal Twist in your daily stretching routine, especially if you experience stiffness or tension in your back.

The Seated Spinal Twist is a simple yet effective way to enhance spinal mobility and overall well-being. As with any stretch, it's important to listen to your body and avoid pushing into pain. Regular practice can contribute to better flexibility, improved posture, and a more balanced body.

Seated Forward Bend

The Seated Forward Bend is a gentle stretching exercise that primarily targets the lower back and hamstrings. It's an excellent choice for improving flexibility in these areas and can also help in relieving tension and stress. This exercise is particularly beneficial for those who spend long hours sitting, as it helps counteract the effects of prolonged sedentary activities.

Instructions for Seated Forward Bend

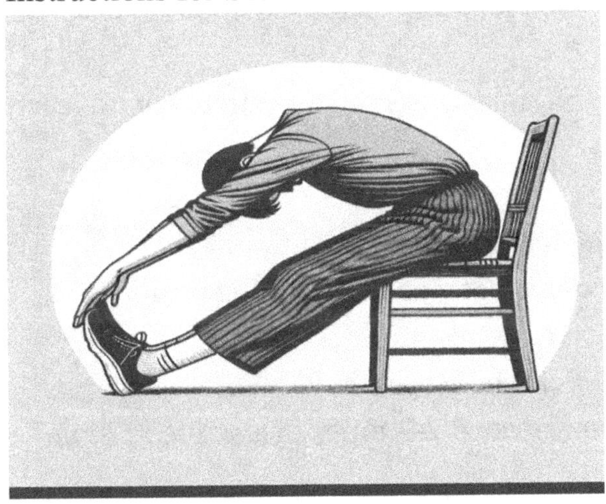

1. Starting Position:

- Sit in a chair with your feet flat on the floor.
- Keep your back straight and hands resting on your thighs.

2. Performing the Exercise:
- Slowly bend forward from your hips, extending your arms towards your feet.
- Keep your head relaxed and facing towards your knees.
- Go as far as you can comfortably, feeling a gentle stretch in your back and legs.

3. Holding the Pose:
- Hold the forward bend position for 15-30 seconds.
- Focus on relaxing into the stretch with each exhale.

4. Returning to Starting Position:
- Slowly come back up to the sitting position.

Number of Sets and Repetitions
- Perform this stretch 2-3 times in a single session.

Frequency

- Include the Seated Forward Bend in your daily stretching routine, especially after long periods of sitting.

The Seated Forward Bend is a simple yet effective way to enhance flexibility and reduce tension in the lower body. It's important to move into and out of the stretch gently and avoid any jerky movements. Regular practice can contribute to better flexibility, improved posture, and overall well-being.

Neck and Shoulder Stretch
The Neck and Shoulder Stretch is an essential exercise for relieving tension in the neck and shoulder areas. This stretch is particularly beneficial for those who experience stiffness due to prolonged sitting, stress, or poor posture. It helps in improving flexibility and can reduce discomfort in the neck and shoulders.

Instructions for Neck and Shoulder Stretch

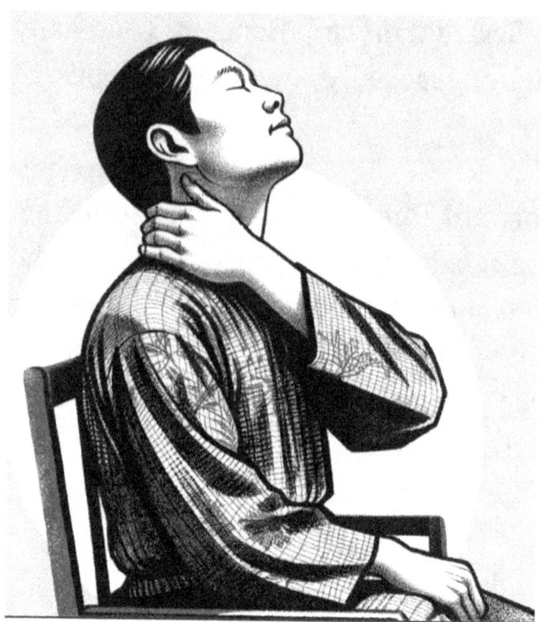

1. Starting Position:

- Sit in a chair with your back straight and feet flat on the floor.

- Keep one hand resting on your thigh or holding onto the chair.

2. Performing the Stretch:

- Gently tilt your head to one side, bringing your ear towards the shoulder.

- Keep the opposite shoulder relaxed and down.

- For a deeper stretch, gently place your hand on the side of your neck or head, applying slight pressure.

3. Holding the Stretch:
- Hold the stretch for 15-30 seconds, breathing deeply and steadily.

4. Switching Sides:
- Carefully release the stretch and repeat on the other side.

Number of Sets and Repetitions
- Beginners: Perform the stretch once on each side.
- Intermediate and Advanced: Repeat the stretch 2-3 times on each side.

Frequency
- Include the Neck and Shoulder Stretch in your daily routine, especially if you work at a desk or experience neck stiffness.

Regular practice of this stretch can lead to increased flexibility in the neck and shoulders, reduced tension, and improved posture. It's a simple yet effective exercise that can be done at your desk or in any seated position.

Chair Warrior I Pose

Chair Warrior I Pose, adapted from the traditional Warrior I pose, is a seated exercise that focuses on enhancing hip flexibility, strengthening the legs, and engaging the upper body. This pose is excellent for stretching the hip flexors, improving leg strength, and promoting overall balance and concentration.

Instructions for Chair Warrior I Pose

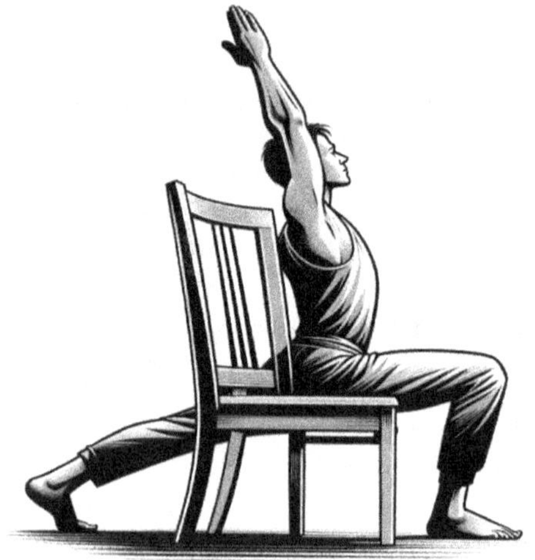

1. Starting Position:
   - Sit in a chair with your feet flat on the floor.
   - Position one foot flat on the floor, knee bent, and extend the other leg straight back, heel lifted.

2. Getting into the Pose:

- Reach your arms overhead, palms facing each other or touching.

- Keep your arms straight and create a long line from the extended back leg through the fingertips.

- Focus on opening your chest and keeping your shoulders relaxed.

3. Holding the Pose:

- Hold the stance for 15-30 seconds, maintaining steady breathing.

- Keep your upper body lifted and your gaze forward.

4. Switching Sides:

- Carefully release the pose and repeat on the other side, switching the position of your legs.

Number of Sets and Repetitions
- Perform the pose once on each side.

Frequency
- Include Chair Warrior I Pose in your daily stretching routine, especially if you're looking to improve hip flexibility and leg strength.

Chair Warrior I Pose is a versatile and beneficial exercise that can be adapted to suit various fitness levels. It's an excellent way to integrate a yoga-inspired movement into your routine, promoting flexibility, strength, and mental focus. Regular practice can contribute to improved posture and overall well-being.

Chair Warrior II Pose

Chair Warrior II Pose is a seated adaptation of the traditional Warrior II pose, focusing on stretching the hips, thighs, and engaging the shoulders. This pose is excellent for improving lower body strength, enhancing upper body posture, and promoting concentration and balance.

Instructions for Chair Warrior II Pose

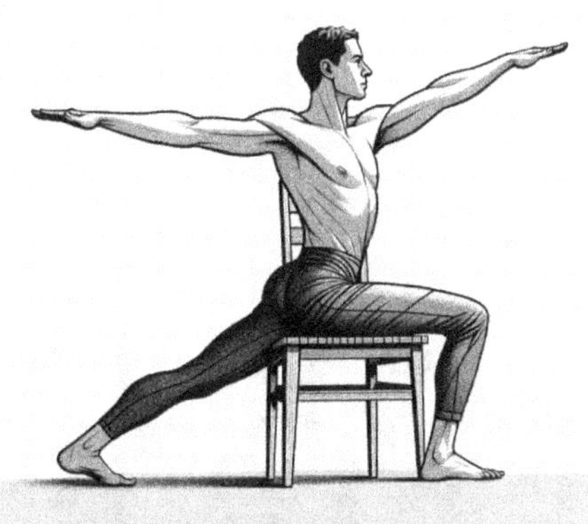

1. Starting Position:

- Sit in a chair with your feet flat on the floor.

- Extend one leg out to the side with the foot flat on the floor, and bend the other knee so the foot is flat and facing forward.

2. Getting into the Pose:

- Extend your arms out to the sides at shoulder height, palms facing down.

- Turn your torso to face the same direction as the bent knee.

- Look over the hand that is on the same side as the bent knee.

3. Holding the Pose:

- Hold the pose for 15-30 seconds, breathing deeply and maintaining focus.
 - Keep your shoulders relaxed and your arms strong.

4. Switching Sides:
 - Carefully release the pose and repeat on the other side, switching the position of your legs and arms.

Number of Sets and Repetitions
- - Beginners: Hold the pose for 10-15 seconds on each side, 1 set.
- - Intermediate: Hold for 20-30 seconds on each side, 1-2 sets.
- - Advanced: Hold for up to 45 seconds on each side, 2-3 sets.

Frequency
- Include Chair Warrior II Pose in your stretching or yoga routine, ideally 2-3 times a week.

Chair Warrior II Pose is a powerful exercise that not only strengthens the body but also helps in centering the mind. It's a wonderful way to integrate a dynamic stretch into your routine, promoting flexibility, strength, and mental clarity. Improved general well-being can result from consistent practice.

Seated Side Stretch

The Seated Side Stretch is a gentle exercise aimed at stretching the oblique muscles and enhancing lateral flexibility. This stretch is beneficial for opening up the side of the body, improving ribcage mobility, and alleviating tightness in the shoulders and neck. It's a fantastic stretch for those who spend a lot of time sitting or wish to improve their overall flexibility.

Instructions for Seated Side Stretch

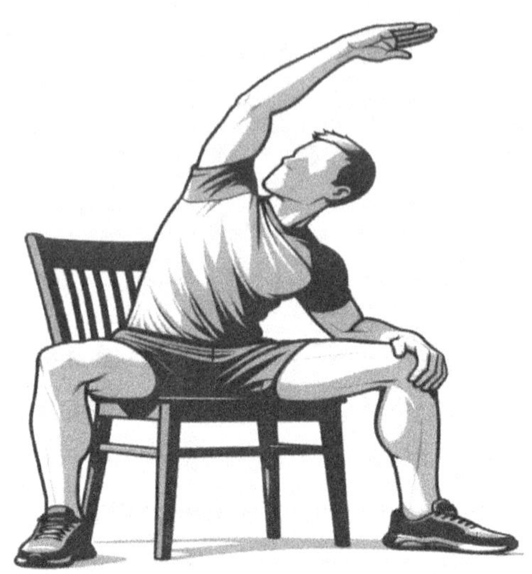

1. Starting Position:

   - Sit in a chair with your feet flat on the floor and your back straight.

   - Keep one hand resting on your thigh or holding onto the side of the chair for support.

2. Performing the Stretch:

   - Extend your other arm overhead and gently lean to the opposite side.

   - Keep your arm close to your ear and focus on creating a long line from your fingertips down to your hips.

- Feel a gentle stretch along the side of your body.

3. Holding the Stretch:
- Hold the stretch for 15-30 seconds, breathing deeply and steadily.
- Keep your posture upright and avoid collapsing forward.

4. Returning to Starting Position and Switching Sides:
- Gently come back to the center and repeat the stretch on the other side.

Number of Sets and Repetitions
- Perform the stretch once on each side.

Frequency
- Include the Seated Side Stretch in your daily stretching routine, especially if you experience tightness in your sides or back.

The Seated Side Stretch is a simple yet effective way to enhance flexibility and reduce tension in the upper body. It's important to perform this stretch gently and avoid any jerky movements. Regular practice can contribute to improved posture and overall well-being.

CHAPTER 7: CARDIO EXERCISES

Chair Star Reach

The Chair Star Reach is a stretching exercise that involves extending the arms and legs outward while seated to form a star shape. This exercise engages the entire body, focusing on stretching the arms, legs, and torso. It's beneficial for enhancing overall flexibility and can help in relieving tension throughout the body.

Instructions for Chair Star Reach

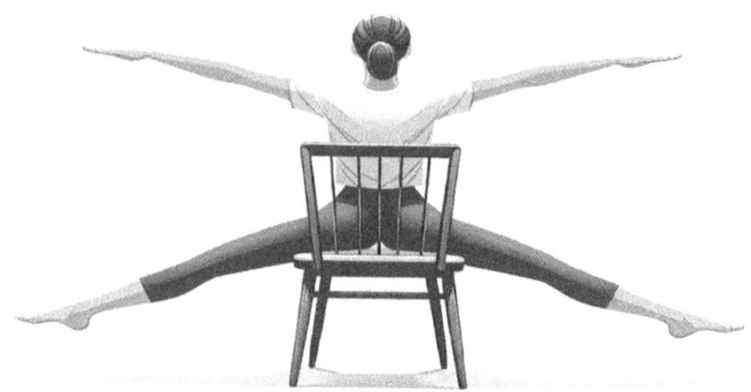

1. Starting Position:

   - Sit in a chair with your back straight and feet flat on the floor.

   - Keep your hands on your thighs or the sides of the chair.

2. Performing the Exercise:

   - Extend your arms and legs outward as far as comfortable to form a star shape.

   - Reach out with your fingertips and toes, stretching as wide as possible.

   - Keep your back straight and focus on maintaining balance.

3. Holding the Stretch:
  - Hold the star shape for 10-15 seconds, breathing deeply and steadily.

4. Returning to Starting Position:
  - Gently bring your arms and legs back to the starting position.

Number of Sets and Repetitions
  - - Beginners: Perform the stretch once, holding for 10-15 seconds.
  - - Intermediate: Hold for 15-20 seconds, repeating 1-2 times.
  - - Advanced: Hold for 20-30 seconds, repeating 2-3 times.

Frequency
- Include the Chair Star Reach in your daily stretching routine, especially if you're looking to improve overall body flexibility.

The Chair Star Reach is a simple and effective way to stretch multiple muscle groups simultaneously. It's a versatile exercise that can be adapted to suit various fitness levels and is particularly useful for those who spend a lot of time sitting. Regular practice can contribute to improved flexibility and overall well-being.

Chair Mountain Climbers

Chair Mountain Climbers are a modified version of the classic mountain climber exercise, adapted for chair use. This version provides a lower-impact alternative while still targeting the core, legs, and improving cardiovascular endurance. It's an excellent exercise for increasing heart rate, strengthening the core, and enhancing leg muscle endurance.

Instructions for Chair Mountain Climbers

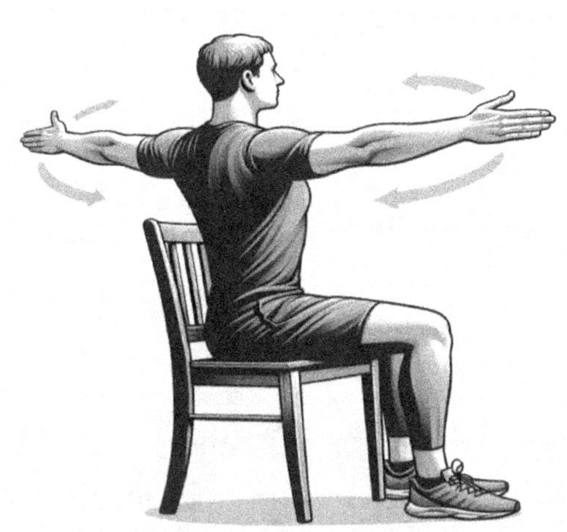

1. Starting Position:

- Stand facing the chair and place your hands on the seat for support.

- Extend your legs back so your body forms a straight line, similar to a plank position.

2. Performing the Exercise:

- Draw one knee towards your chest, keeping the other leg extended back.

- Quickly switch legs, extending the bent leg back and drawing the other knee towards your chest.

- Continue alternating legs in a controlled, rhythmic motion.

3. Repetitions and Sets:

- - Beginners: Perform for 20-30 seconds, 1-2 sets.
- - Intermediate: Perform for 30-45 seconds, 2-3 sets.
- - Advanced: Perform for 45-60 seconds, 3-4 sets.

Frequency

- Include Chair Mountain Climbers in your cardiovascular or core workout routine, ideally 2-3 times a week.

Chair Mountain Climbers are a dynamic and effective way to engage multiple muscle groups and increase your heart rate. They can be easily incorporated into any fitness routine and offer a convenient way to get a cardiovascular workout without needing a lot of space or equipment. Regular practice can lead to improved cardiovascular health, core strength, and overall physical endurance.

Seated Bicycle Legs

Seated Bicycle Legs is a low-impact cardiovascular and strength exercise, adapted from the traditional bicycle crunch. Performed while seated, it targets the core, hip flexors, and leg muscles. This exercise is excellent for improving lower body mobility and core strength, making it suitable for those who prefer seated workouts.

Instructions for Seated Bicycle Legs

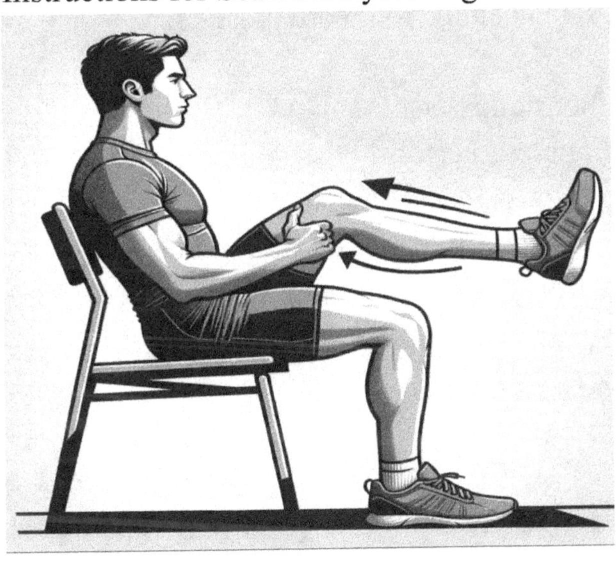

1. Starting Position:
   - Sit in a chair with your back straight and feet flat on the floor.

- Place your hands on your thighs or hold onto the sides of the chair for balance.

2. Performing the Exercise:
   - Extend one leg out, straightening it as much as possible.
   - Then draw the knee back in towards your chest.
   - Alternate between legs, simulating a bicycle pedaling motion.
   - Keep your movements smooth and controlled, focusing on engaging your core muscles.

3. Repetitions and Sets:
   - Beginners: Perform the motion for 30-60 seconds, 1-2 sets.
   - Intermediate: Continue for 1-2 minutes, 2-3 sets.
   - Advanced: Aim for 2-3 minutes or more, 3-4 sets.

Frequency
- Include Seated Bicycle Legs in your routine 2-3 times a week, especially as part of a low-impact cardiovascular or core workout.

Seated Bicycle Legs offer a practical and effective way to engage in cardiovascular and core strengthening exercises. They are particularly beneficial for those looking for a safe and accessible way to maintain fitness, especially for individuals with limited mobility or those who spend a lot of time sitting. Regular practice can lead to improved core strength, leg muscle endurance, and overall cardiovascular health.

Chair Running

Chair Running is a dynamic, low-impact cardiovascular exercise that simulates the motion of running while seated. This exercise is excellent for improving circulation and endurance, particularly targeting the legs and arms. It's ideal for those who are looking for an effective cardio workout without the strain of high-impact movements.

Instructions for Chair Running

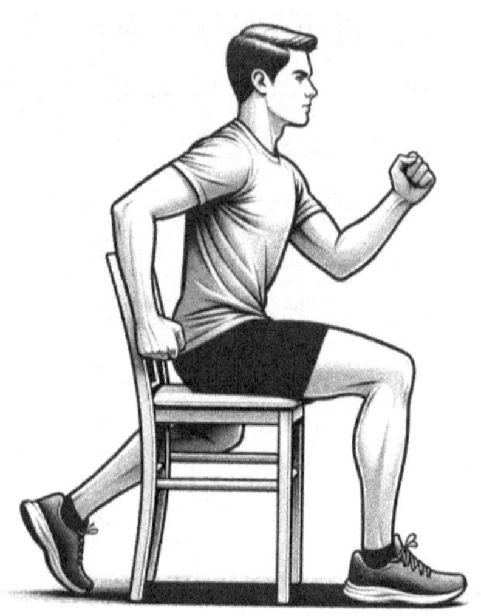

1. Starting Position:

   - Sit in a chair with your back straight and feet flat on the floor.

   - Place your hands by your sides or on your thighs.

2. Performing the Exercise:

   - Begin by lifting your knees alternately, as if running in place.

   - Simultaneously move your arms back and forth, mirroring the movement of your legs.

   - Maintain an upright posture and focus on engaging your core for balance.

3. Repetitions and Sets:

- - Beginners: Perform the running motion for 30-60 seconds, 1-2 sets.
- - Intermediate: Continue for 1-2 minutes, 2-3 sets.
- - Advanced: Aim for 2-3 minutes or more, 3-4 sets.

Frequency
- Include Chair Running in your cardiovascular workout routine, ideally 2-3 times a week.

Chair Running provides an excellent cardio workout and can be especially beneficial for improving lower body strength and cardiovascular health. It's a convenient and safe exercise for people of all ages and fitness levels, offering a practical way to stay active, particularly for those with limited mobility or space.

Seated Jacks

Seated Jacks are a low-impact cardiovascular exercise, adapted from the traditional jumping jack for seated practice. This exercise provides a great way to increase heart rate and improve circulation, targeting both the arms and legs. It's especially beneficial for individuals looking for a gentle yet effective cardio workout without the stress of standing exercises.

Instructions for Seated Jacks

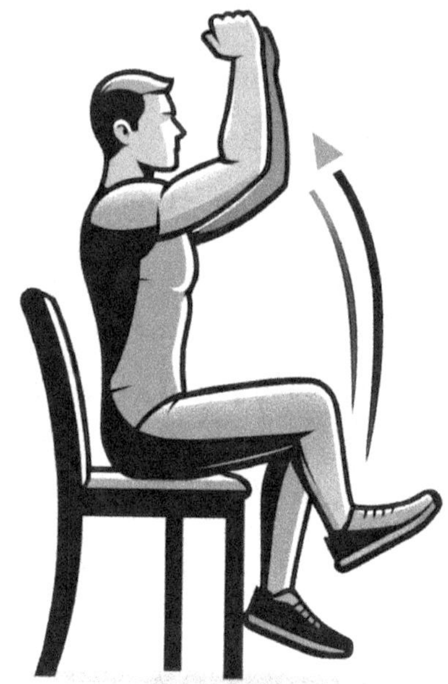

1. Starting Position:
   - Sit in a chair with your back straight and feet flat on the floor.
   - Place your hands by your sides.

2. Performing the Exercise:

- Simultaneously move your arms up and down from the sides to above your head.

- At the same time, extend and bring your legs in and out to the sides, mimicking the movement of a traditional jumping jack.

- Maintain an upright posture throughout the exercise.

3. Repetitions and Sets:

- - Beginners: Perform for 20-30 seconds, 1-2 sets.
- - Intermediate: Perform for 30-45 seconds, 2-3 sets.
- - Advanced: Perform for 45-60 seconds, 3-4 sets.

Frequency

- Include Seated Jacks in your cardiovascular workout routine, ideally 2-3 times a week.

Seated Jacks offer an excellent way to engage in cardiovascular activity, particularly for those who prefer or need low-impact exercises. Regular practice can lead to improved cardiovascular health, increased energy levels, and overall enhanced physical fitness.

Seated Arm Circles

Seated Arm Circles are a versatile exercise ideal for improving shoulder mobility and arm strength. This seated adaptation makes it accessible for individuals of all fitness levels, especially those who may have limited standing mobility. It's an effective way to warm up the shoulders and arms, and can also help in relieving tension in the upper body.

Instructions for Seated Arm Circles

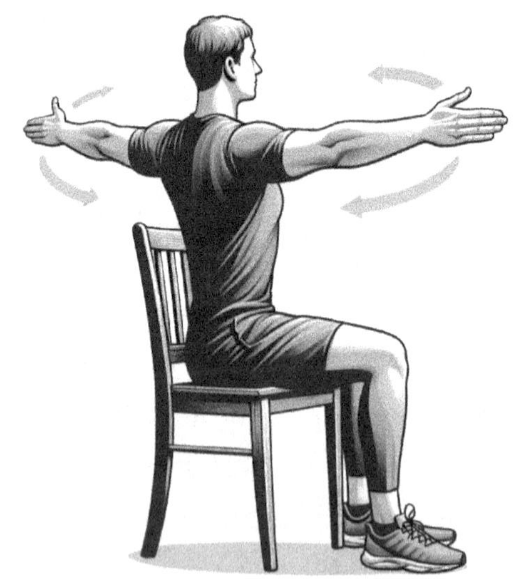

1. Starting Position:
- Sit in a chair with your back straight and feet flat on the floor.
- Extend your arms out to the sides at shoulder height.

2. Performing the Exercise:
- Rotate your arms in small circles, starting in a forward direction.
- Keep your movements controlled and focus on using your shoulder muscles.
- After a set number of circles, reverse the direction and rotate your arms backward.

3. Repetitions and Sets:
- Beginners: Perform 10-15 circles in each direction, 1 set.
- Intermediate: Perform 15-20 circles in each direction, 2 sets.
- Advanced: Perform 20-25 circles in each direction, 3 sets.

Frequency
- Include Seated Arm Circles in your daily routine or workout regimen, particularly as a warm-up for upper body exercises.

Seated Arm Circles are excellent for maintaining shoulder health, enhancing upper body mobility, and can be done anywhere, making them a convenient exercise for those with a sedentary lifestyle. Regular practice can lead to improved mobility and reduced stiffness in the shoulders and arms.

CHAPTER 8: MOBILITY, POSTURE, AND BALANCE

Seated Ankle Flex and Point

Seated Ankle Flex and Point is a simple yet effective exercise for strengthening the muscles in the lower leg and improving ankle flexibility. This exercise is particularly beneficial for those who may have limited mobility or spend extended periods sitting, as it helps in maintaining ankle movement and circulation.

Instructions for Seated Ankle Flex and Point

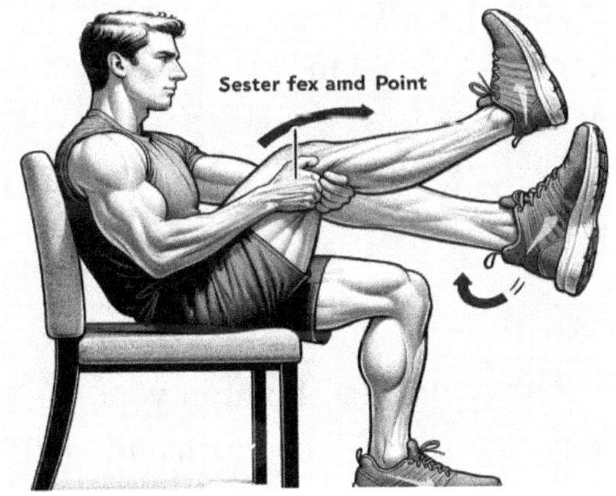

1. Starting Position:

- Sit in a chair with your back straight and feet flat on the floor.

- Extend one leg out in front of you, with the foot off the ground.

2. Performing the Exercise:

- Alternate between flexing your ankle (pulling the toes towards the shin) and pointing your toes away.

- Keep the movements controlled and focused on the ankle joint.

- Ensure your leg remains straight throughout the exercise.

3. Repetitions and Sets:

- Beginners: Perform 10-15 flexes and points per foot, 1-2 sets.

- Intermediate: Perform 15-20 flexes and points per foot, 2-3 sets.

- Advanced: Perform 20-25 flexes and points per foot, 3-4 sets.

Frequency

- Include Seated Ankle Flex and Point in your daily routine, especially as a way to maintain ankle mobility and prevent stiffness.

This exercise is excellent for promoting foot and ankle health, particularly for individuals who are less active or have restrictions in standing and walking. Regular practice can lead to improved flexibility in the ankles, better circulation in the lower extremities, and overall enhanced foot health.

Chair Leg Lifts and Holds

Chair Leg Lifts and Holds are an effective exercise for strengthening the leg muscles and improving core stability. This seated exercise is ideal for targeting the thigh muscles and the core, and it's beneficial for enhancing muscle endurance and balance.

Instructions for Chair Leg Lifts and Holds

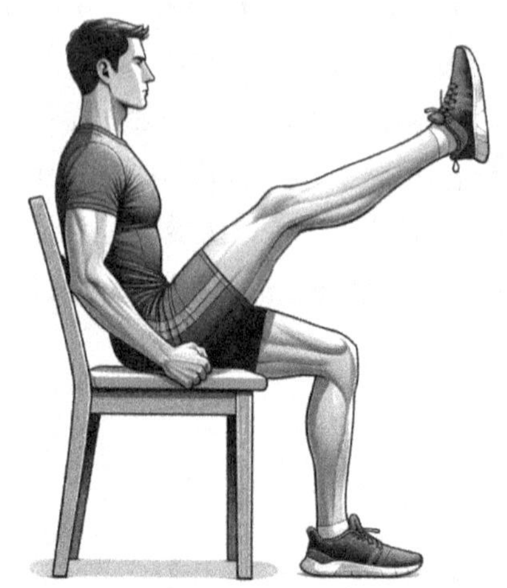

1. Starting Position:

   - Sit in a chair with your back straight and feet flat on the floor.

   - Place your hands on the sides of the chair for support.

2. Performing the Exercise:

   - Lift one leg straight out in front of you, keeping it as straight as possible.

   - Hold the lifted leg in the air, engaging your core and thigh muscles.

   - Maintain a straight back and focused posture.

3. Holding the Position:

- Hold the leg lift for 10-30 seconds, depending on your ability.

4. Repetitions and Sets:
- • - Beginners: Hold for 10 seconds per leg, 1-2 sets.
- • - Intermediate: Hold for 15-20 seconds per leg, 2-3 sets.
- • - Advanced: Hold for 20-30 seconds per leg, 3-4 sets.

Frequency
- Include Chair Leg Lifts and Holds in your routine 2-3 times a week for optimal results.

Chair Leg Lifts and Holds are excellent for improving lower body strength and core stability. They can be easily incorporated into any fitness routine and are especially beneficial for those who spend a lot of time sitting. Regular practice can lead to improved leg muscle strength, better balance, and enhanced core stability.

Seated Hip Circles

Seated Hip Circles are an excellent exercise for improving hip mobility and flexibility. This seated exercise is particularly beneficial for those who spend long periods sitting or who have limited mobility. It helps in engaging and loosening the hip flexors and lower back, promoting better movement and reducing stiffness.

Instructions for Seated Hip Circles

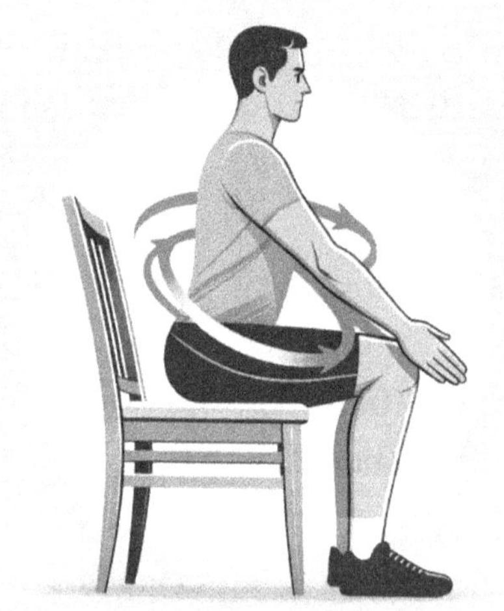

1. Starting Position:
   - Sit in a chair with your back straight and feet flat on the floor.

- Place your hands on your thighs or the sides of the chair for support.

2. Performing the Exercise:
- Begin by rotating your hips in a circular motion, moving them forward, to the side, backward, and then to the other side.
- Keep the movement smooth and controlled.
- Focus on using your core and hip muscles to perform the circles.

3. Repetitions and Sets:
- Beginners: Perform 5-10 circles in each direction, 1-2 sets.
- Intermediate: Perform 10-15 circles in each direction, 2-3 sets.
- Advanced: Perform 15-20 circles in each direction, 3-4 sets.

Frequency
- Include Seated Hip Circles in your daily routine, especially if you're looking to improve hip flexibility and reduce stiffness.

Seated Hip Circles are a simple yet effective way to maintain hip health. They're a practical exercise for people of all ages and fitness levels and can be easily incorporated into any daily routine. Regular practice can lead to improved hip mobility, reduced tension, and better overall physical health.

Chair Child's Pose

Chair Child's Pose is a seated adaptation of the traditional Child's Pose in yoga. This version is designed to provide similar benefits, focusing on relaxing the back and shoulders. It's a gentle stretch that can help alleviate tension and promote relaxation, making it suitable for all levels of fitness.

Instructions for Chair Child's Pose

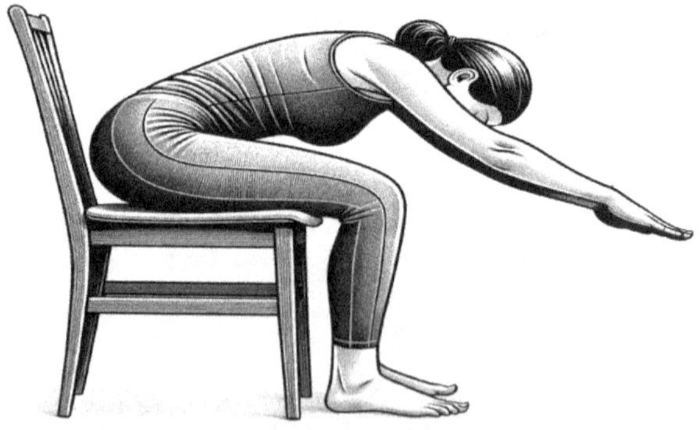

1. Starting Position:
   - Sit in a chair with your feet flat on the floor.
   - Keep your back straight and hands resting on your thighs.

2. Performing the Pose:
   - Lean forward, bringing your torso towards your thighs.
   - Extend your arms forward, resting them either on your thighs or reaching towards the ground with palms down.
   - Let your head relax and gently bow it.

3. Holding the Pose:
   - Hold this relaxed position for 1-2 minutes, focusing on deep, steady breaths.
   - Feel the stretch in your back and the relaxation in your shoulders.

4. Frequency:
   - Practice Chair Child's Pose as needed, especially when seeking moments of relaxation or during a yoga sequence.

Chair Child's Pose is excellent for times of stress or after long periods of sitting. It offers a moment of calm and is an easy way to introduce gentle stretching into your daily routine. Regular practice can contribute to reduced tension in the back and shoulders, improved posture, and overall well-being.

Seated Mountain Pose

Seated Mountain Pose, adapted from the traditional yoga Mountain Pose, is a practice of grounding and centering while seated. This pose is excellent for improving posture, enhancing breathing, and cultivating mental focus. It's a fundamental pose that can be easily integrated into daily routines or as part of a seated yoga practice.

Instructions for Seated Mountain Pose

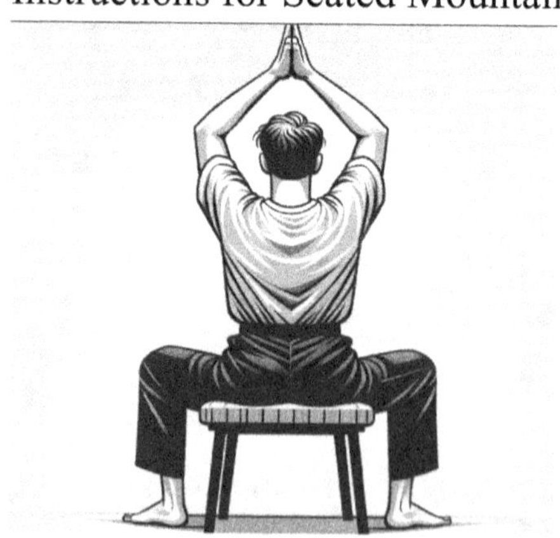

1. Starting Position:

- Sit in a chair with your back straight and feet flat on the floor, legs hip-width apart.

2. Performing the Pose:
   - Rest your hands on your thighs or raise them above your head with palms facing each other.
   - Keep your back straight, shoulders relaxed, and gaze forward.
   - Engage your core slightly to maintain an upright posture.

3. Holding the Pose:
   - Hold this position for 1-2 minutes, focusing on your breath and maintaining steady, deep breaths.

4. Frequency:
   - Practice Seated Mountain Pose daily, especially as part of a seated yoga sequence or when seeking moments of relaxation and focus.

Seated Mountain Pose is beneficial for anyone seeking to improve their posture and find a moment of calm in their day. It's a versatile pose that encourages mindfulness and body awareness, making it ideal for both beginners and experienced yoga practitioners. Regular practice can contribute to better posture, reduced stress, and overall well-being.

Chair Tree Pose

Chair Tree Pose is a seated adaptation of the traditional Tree Pose in yoga. This version is performed while seated in a chair, making it more accessible and suitable for those who might have difficulty standing. The pose focuses on improving balance and stability, and is excellent for enhancing concentration and posture.

Instructions for Chair Tree Pose

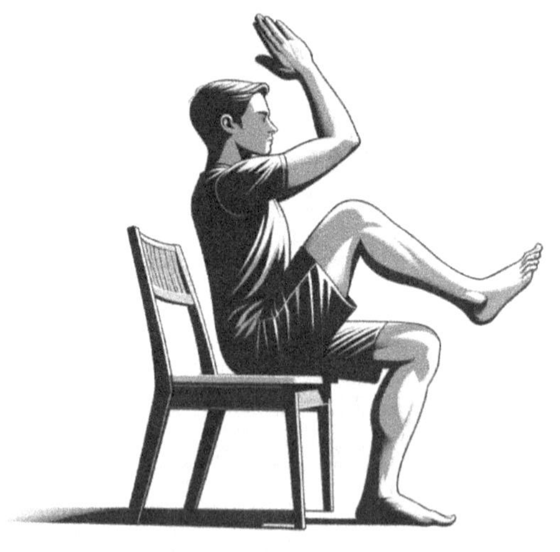

1. Starting Position:

- Sit in a chair with your back straight and feet flat on the floor.

- Maintain an upright posture throughout the exercise.

2. Performing the Pose:

- Place the sole of one foot on the inner thigh of the opposite leg, avoiding the knee joint.

- Keep the raised knee pointing out to the side.

- For balance, place your hands on your lap or bring them together in a prayer position at your chest or above your head.

3. Holding the Pose:

- Hold the pose for 15-30 seconds, focusing on maintaining your balance and a steady breathing pattern.

4. Switching Sides:

- Carefully release the pose and repeat on the other side.

Repetitions and Sets:
- Perform the pose once on each side.

- For a more challenging variation, try holding the pose for a longer duration or closing your eyes to enhance balance skills.

Frequency:
- Include the Chair Tree Pose in your daily routine or as part of a yoga or balance training session.

Chair Tree Pose is beneficial for individuals of all ages and fitness levels, particularly for those seeking a gentle yet effective way to improve balance and concentration. Regular practice can contribute to better posture and overall well-being.

THE CHAIR YOGA 28-CHALLENGE

Creating a 28-day challenge with morning and evening sessions is a great way to establish a consistent practice and see progressive benefits.

Day 1 - Day 7: Introduction and Foundation Building

Day 8 - Day 14: Flexibility and Strength Focus

Day 15 - Day 21: Balance and Core Strengthening

Day 22 - Day 28: Integration and Advanced Practice

Notes for the Challenge:
- - Each session should start with a few minutes of deep breathing to center and prepare the body.
- - Conclude each session with a few minutes of relaxation, sitting comfortably or doing a seated meditation.

- - Listen to your body and modify poses as needed. The goal is to challenge yourself but remain comfortable and free from pain.
- - Stay hydrated and follow a balanced diet to complement your yoga practice.
- - Reflect on your experience at the end of each week and adjust the intensity as needed.

This 28-day challenge is designed to progressively build your strength, flexibility, balance, and overall well-being. By dedicating time each morning and evening to your practice, you'll be able to fully experience the benefits of chair yoga.

<u>Week 1: Introduction and Foundation Building</u>

Day 1:

- Morning: Seated Mountain Pose (5 minutes), Seated Forward Bend (3 repetitions)
- Evening: Seated Cat-Cow Stretch (5 minutes), Seated Twist (3 repetitions each side)

Day 2:
- Morning: Seated Forward Bend (3 repetitions), Seated Cat-Cow Stretch (5 minutes)
- Evening: Seated Twist (3 repetitions each side), Seated Mountain Pose (5 minutes)

Day 3:
- Morning: Seated Cat-Cow Stretch (5 minutes), Seated Twist (3 repetitions each side)
- Evening: Seated Mountain Pose (5 minutes), Seated Forward Bend (3 repetitions)

Day 4:
- Morning: Seated Twist (3 repetitions each side), Seated Mountain Pose (5 minutes)
- Evening: Seated Forward Bend (3 repetitions), Seated Cat-Cow Stretch (5 minutes)

Day 5:
- Morning: Seated Mountain Pose (5 minutes), Seated Cat-Cow Stretch (5 minutes)

- Evening: Seated Forward Bend (3 repetitions), Seated Twist (3 repetitions each side)

Day 6:
- Morning: Seated Forward Bend (3 repetitions), Seated Twist (3 repetitions each side)
- Evening: Seated Cat-Cow Stretch (5 minutes), Seated Mountain Pose (5 minutes)

Day 7:
- Morning: Seated Cat-Cow Stretch (5 minutes), Seated Mountain Pose (5 minutes)
- Evening: Seated Twist (3 repetitions each side), Seated Forward Bend (3 repetitions)

Daily Guidelines:
- Start each session with a minute of deep, relaxed breathing to center yourself.
- Focus on the smooth transition between poses and maintaining deep, steady breathing throughout.
- End each session with a minute of relaxation, either in a comfortable seated position or with a brief meditation to reflect on your practice.

- Stay mindful of your body's responses and make modifications as needed for comfort and safety.
- Consistency is key; try to practice at the same time each morning and evening to establish a routine.

This first week is designed to introduce you to the fundamentals of chair yoga, focusing on building a foundation in flexibility, balance, and mindful breathing.

Week 2: Flexibility and Building strength

Day 8 to Day 14: Enhancing Flexibility and Building Strength

Day 8:
- Morning: Seated Hip Opener
 (3 minutes each side), Seated Tree Pose (2 minutes each side)
- Evening: Chair Leg Lifts and Holds (10 repetitions each leg), Seated Twist (3 repetitions each side)

Day 9:

- Morning: Seated Warrior I (2 minutes each side), Seated Forward Bend (3 repetitions)
- Evening: Seated Cat-Cow Stretch (5 minutes), Seated Mountain Pose (5 minutes)

Day 10:
- Morning: Seated Tree Pose (2 minutes each side), Seated Hip Circles (3 minutes each side)
- Evening: Seated Twist (3 repetitions each side), Chair Leg Lifts and Holds (10 repetitions each leg)

Day 11:
- Morning: Seated Forward Bend (3 repetitions), Seated Warrior I (2 minutes each side)
- Evening: Seated Mountain Pose (5 minutes), Seated Cat-Cow Stretch (5 minutes)

Day 12:
- Morning: Chair Leg Lifts and Holds (10 repetitions each leg), Seated Hip Circles (3 minutes each side)
- Evening: Seated Tree Pose (2 minutes each side), Seated Twist (3 repetitions each side)

Day 13:
- Morning: Seated Warrior I (2 minutes each side), Seated Forward Bend (3 repetitions)

- Evening: Seated Cat-Cow Stretch (5 minutes), Seated Mountain Pose (5 minutes)

Day 14:
- Morning: Seated Tree Pose (2 minutes each side), Chair Leg Lifts and Holds (10 repetitions each leg)
- Evening: Seated Hip Circles (3 minutes each side), Seated Twist (3 repetitions each side)

Weekly Focus:
- This week aims to enhance flexibility and build strength, particularly in the lower body and core.
- Pay attention to how your body feels during each pose and make adjustments as needed.
- Keep your breath steady and deep, especially during longer holds.
- Finish each session with a moment of relaxation and reflection, appreciating the progress you're making.

Maintain consistency in your practice, and you'll start to notice improvements in your flexibility, balance, and overall strength. Remember, it's not about perfection but progress.

Week 3: Balance, posture and mobility

Day 15 to Day 21: Focusing on Balance and Core Strengthening

Day 15:
- Morning: Seated Twist (2 minutes each side), Chair Pigeon Pose (2 minutes each side)
- Evening: Seated Forward Bend (4 repetitions), Seated Cat-Cow Stretch (5 minutes)

Day 16:
- Morning: Chair Leg Lifts and Holds (12 repetitions each leg), Seated Mountain Pose (5 minutes)
- Evening: Seated Tree Pose (2 minutes each side), Seated Hip Circles (3 minutes each side)

Day 17:

- Morning: Seated Warrior I (2 minutes each side), Seated Twist (2 minutes each side)
- Evening: Chair Pigeon Pose (2 minutes each side), Seated Cat-Cow Stretch (5 minutes)

Day 18:
- Morning: Seated Hip Circles (3 minutes each side), Seated Forward Bend (4 repetitions)
- Evening: Seated Mountain Pose (5 minutes), Chair Leg Lifts and Holds (12 repetitions each leg)

Day 19:
- Morning: Seated Tree Pose (2 minutes each side), Chair Pigeon Pose (2 minutes each side)
- Evening: Seated Twist (2 minutes each side), Seated Warrior I (2 minutes each side)

Day 20:
- Morning: Seated Cat-Cow Stretch (5 minutes), Seated Forward Bend (4 repetitions)
- Evening: Chair Leg Lifts and Holds (12 repetitions each leg), Seated Mountain Pose (5 minutes)

Day 21:
- Morning: Seated Warrior I (2 minutes each side), Seated Hip Circles (3 minutes each side)

- Evening: Seated Tree Pose (2 minutes each side), Chair Pigeon Pose (2 minutes each side)

Weekly Focus:
- This week emphasizes balance and core strength, key components for overall stability and posture.
- Each morning session is designed to activate and energize your body for the day.
- The evening sessions focus on relaxation and deeper stretching to improve flexibility.
- Continue to breathe deeply and mindfully during each exercise, focusing on your body's alignment and balance.
- End each session with a brief period of relaxation or meditation, reflecting on your body's sensations and progress.

Keep up the dedication to your practice, and you'll likely see improvements in your core stability, balance, and overall mindfulness. Remember, consistency is crucial to gaining the full benefits of chair yoga.

Week 4: Integration and Advanced Practice

Day 22 to Day 28: Advanced Integration and Practice Enhancement

Day 22:
- Morning: Seated Warrior I (3 minutes each side), Chair Pigeon Pose (2 minutes each side)
- Evening: Seated Hip Circles (4 minutes each side), Seated Twist (3 repetitions each side)

Day 23:
- Morning: Chair Leg Lifts and Holds (15 repetitions each leg), Seated Tree Pose (3 minutes each side)
- Evening: Seated Forward Bend (5 repetitions), Seated Cat-Cow Stretch (6 minutes)

Day 24:
- Morning: Seated Mountain Pose (6 minutes), Seated Twist (3 minutes each side)
- Evening: Chair Pigeon Pose (3 minutes each side), Seated Warrior I (3 minutes each side)

Day 25:
- Morning: Seated Forward Bend (5 repetitions), Seated Hip Circles (4 minutes each side)
- Evening: Seated Cat-Cow Stretch (6 minutes), Chair Leg Lifts and Holds (15 repetitions each leg)

Day 26:
- Morning: Seated Tree Pose (3 minutes each side), Seated Warrior I (3 minutes each side)
- Evening: Seated Twist (3 minutes each side), Chair Pigeon Pose (3 minutes each side)

Day 27:
- Morning: Chair Leg Lifts and Holds (15 repetitions each leg), Seated Mountain Pose (6 minutes)
- Evening: Seated Hip Circles (4 minutes each side), Seated Forward Bend (5 repetitions)

Day 28:
- Morning: Seated Cat-Cow Stretch (6 minutes), Seated Tree Pose (3 minutes each side)
- Evening: Chair Pigeon Pose (3 minutes each side), Seated Warrior I (3 minutes each side)

Weekly Focus:

- This final week is about integrating everything you've learned and practiced. The focus is on longer holds and deeper stretches to enhance flexibility, strength, and mindfulness.
- Pay attention to the smoothness of your transitions between poses and the depth of your breathing.
- Use this week to observe any changes in your flexibility, strength, balance, and overall well-being.
- End each session with a few minutes of relaxation or meditation, acknowledging your progress and the dedication you've shown throughout this challenge.

Congratulations on completing the 28-day chair yoga challenge! You've made a significant commitment to your physical and mental health. Continue to incorporate these practices into your daily routine to maintain and further the benefits you've achieved.

During the course of these exercises feel free to TWEAK the exercises or change a certain exercise with the one you prefer if the challenge is not comfortable.

CHAIR YOGA WEEKLY CHALLENGE

WEEKLY MOTIVATION: "STRENGTH DOES NOT COME FROM PHYSICAL CAPACITY. IT COMES FROM AN INDOMITABLE WIGS." - MAHARMA GANDHI

	MORNING	AFTERNOON	EVENING
MON			
TUES			
WED			
THURS			
FRI			
SAT			

NOTE ON NEW WEEKLY DISCOVERIES

CHAIR YOGA WEEKLY CHALLENGE

WEEKLY MOTIVATION: "DO NOT COUNT THE DAYS; MAKE THE DAYS COUNT." - MUHAMMAD ABL.

	MORNING	AFTERNOON	EVENING
MON			
TUES			
WED			
THURS			
FRI			
SAT			

NOTE ON NEW WEEKLY DISCOVERIES

CHAIR YOGA WEEKLY CHALLENGE

WEEKLY MOTIVATION: "THE ONLY WAY TO ACHIEVE THE IMPOSSIBLE IS TO BELIEVE IT IS POSSIBLE." - CHARLES KINGSLEIGH

	MORNING	AFTERNOON	EVENING
MON			
TUES			
WED			
THURS			
FRI			
SAT			

NOTE ON NEW WEEKLY DISCOVERIES

MEAL PLAN(14-DAYS)

I have designed these 15 recipes designed to complement your chair yoga routine, providing the nourishment and energy needed to support your exercise regimen.

1. Avocado and Egg Toast
   - Whole-grain toast topped with mashed avocado and a poached egg.
   - Ideal for a pre-yoga breakfast, offering a balance of healthy fats, protein, and carbs.

2. Berry Almond Smoothie
   - Blend mixed berries, almond milk, a banana, and a scoop of protein powder.
   - A refreshing post-yoga drink to replenish and energize.

3. Greek Yogurt Parfait
   - Layer Greek yogurt with granola and fresh berries.
   - Provides calcium and protein, perfect for a post-exercise snack.

4. Quinoa Salad
 - Toss cooked quinoa with cherry tomatoes, cucumber, feta cheese, and a lemon-olive oil dressing.
 - A light and nutritious meal for lunch, rich in protein and fiber.

5. Grilled Chicken and Vegetable Stir-Fry
 - Sauté chicken with a mix of your favorite vegetables and a soy-ginger sauce.
 - Ideal for dinner, offering lean protein and a variety of nutrients.

6. Spinach and Banana Protein Smoothie
 - Blend spinach, a banana, almond milk, and a scoop of vanilla protein powder.
 - A quick, nutrient-packed breakfast or snack to fuel your yoga practice.

7. Lentil Soup
 - Simmer lentils with vegetables and spices for a comforting meal.
 - A great source of plant-based protein and fiber, perfect for a post-yoga dinner.

8. Almond Butter and Banana Sandwich

- Whole-grain bread with almond butter and banana slices.
- A satisfying and energy-boosting snack for any time of the day.

9. Hummus and Veggie Wrap
- Spread hummus on a whole-grain wrap and fill with mixed salad greens and sliced vegetables.
- A light yet filling lunch option, providing fiber and essential nutrients.

10. Oatmeal with Nuts and Berries
- Cook oats and top with mixed nuts and fresh berries.
- A hearty breakfast to start your day with sustained energy.

11. Tuna Salad
- Mix canned tuna with light mayo, diced celery, and onion. Serve on a bed of lettuce.
- A protein-rich lunch to support muscle recovery after yoga.

12. Baked Sweet Potato with Grilled Veggies
- Serve a baked sweet potato with a side of grilled bell peppers, zucchini, and onions.

- A nutritious and satisfying dinner, packed with vitamins and minerals.

13. Cottage Cheese with Pineapple
   - Combine cottage cheese with fresh pineapple chunks.
   - A perfect snack for a quick protein and energy boost.

14. Turkey and Avocado Salad
   - Toss diced turkey breast with avocado, mixed greens, and a vinaigrette dressing.
   - A balanced meal for lunch, offering healthy fats, protein, and fiber.

15. Protein Pancakes
   - Make pancakes using protein powder, eggs, and oats. Serve with fresh fruit.
   - A delicious and energizing post-yoga breakfast or brunch.

These recipes are designed to be simple, nutritious, and aligned with the energy needs of your chair yoga exercises. They focus on providing a balance of proteins, healthy fats, and carbohydrates to support your practice and overall well-being.

Incorporating these recipes into your routine alongside chair yoga exercises can optimize your health and wellness goals. Effective use of these recipes.

How to use

1. Pre-Yoga Nutrition:

- Consume light, energizing meals or snacks about 30-60 minutes before your yoga session. Options like the Berry Almond Smoothie or Avocado and Egg Toast provide a good balance of carbohydrates and protein without being too heavy.

- Hydrate well with water or a hydrating smoothie like the Spinach and Banana Protein Smoothie.

2. Post-Yoga Nutrition:

- Within 30 minutes to an hour after your yoga practice, focus on meals rich in protein to aid in muscle recovery. The Grilled Chicken and Vegetable Stir-Fry or Greek Yogurt Parfait are great choices.

- Rehydrate with water or a refreshing beverage like a fruit smoothie.

3. Daily Meals:

- For regular meals, choose recipes that offer a balance of protein, healthy fats, and carbohydrates. The Quinoa Salad, Lentil Soup, or Tuna Salad are excellent for lunch, providing sustained energy for the day.

- Dinner should be wholesome but not too heavy, like the Baked Sweet Potato with Grilled Veggies or Turkey and Avocado Salad, ensuring you don't go to bed feeling overly full.

4. Snacks:

- Healthy snacks like the Cottage Cheese with Pineapple or Almond Butter and Banana Sandwich can be consumed between meals to maintain energy levels and prevent overeating during main meals.

- These snacks are also ideal for those times when you need a quick boost, especially after an intense yoga session.

5. Listen to Your Body:

- Pay attention to your body's hunger and fullness cues. Eat when you're hungry but avoid overeating.

- Adjust portion sizes and meal frequency based on your activity level, yoga intensity, and personal health goals.

6. Hydration:

- Stay hydrated throughout the day, not just during and after your yoga sessions. Water is essential for overall health and aids in digestion and nutrient absorption.

By aligning your nutrition with your chair yoga practice, you can enhance the benefits of the exercises, aid in recovery, and support your overall physical and mental well-being. Remember, consistency in both your exercise and dietary habits is key to achieving the best results.

<u>Meal planner</u>

I have designed a beautiful two-week meal plan that incorporates the provided recipes, specifying pre-workout and post-workout meals to complement your chair yoga sessions.

Week 1:

Day 1:
- Pre-workout: Banana and Almond Butter Smoothie
- Post-workout: Greek Yogurt Parfait

Day 2:
- Pre-workout: Oatmeal with Nuts and Berries
- Post-workout: Tuna Salad

Day 3:
- Pre-workout: Avocado and Egg Toast
- Post-workout: Quinoa Salad

Day 4:
- Pre-workout: Berry Almond Smoothie
- Post-workout: Grilled Chicken and Vegetable Stir-Fry

Day 5:
- Pre-workout: Spinach and Banana Protein
Smoothie
- Post-workout: Lentil Soup

Day 6:
- Pre-workout: Cottage Cheese with Pineapple
- Post-workout: Baked Sweet Potato with Grilled
Veggies

Day 7:
- Pre-workout: Whole Grain Pancakes with Fresh
Fruit
- Post-workout: Turkey and Avocado Salad

Week 2:

Day 8:
- Pre-workout: Scrambled Eggs with Spinach and
Feta
- Post-workout: Hummus and Veggie Wrap

Day 9:
- Pre-workout: Chia Seed Pudding with Berries
- Post-workout: Baked Lemon-Garlic Tilapia with
Quinoa

Day 10:
- Pre-workout: Greek Yogurt with Honey and Nuts
- Post-workout: Stir-Fried Beef with Broccoli and Brown Rice

Day 11:
- Pre-workout: Protein Pancakes with a Banana
- Post-workout: Grilled Pork Tenderloin with Roasted Brussels Sprouts

Day 12:
- Pre-workout: Smoothie with Spinach, Banana, and Almond Milk
- Post-workout: Chicken Caesar Salad

Day 13:
- Pre-workout: Almond Butter and Banana Sandwich
- Post-workout: Quinoa and Black Bean Bowl

Day 14:
- Pre-workout: Overnight Oats with Apples and Cinnamon
- Post-workout: Grilled Shrimp over Mixed Greens Salad

Note:
- Hydrate well with water before and after your workouts.
- Adjust portion sizes according to your appetite and energy needs.
- This meal plan can be modified based on dietary preferences and restrictions.

This two-week meal plan is designed to provide balanced nutrition that supports your chair yoga practice, ensuring you have the energy for your workouts and the right nutrients for recovery.

CONCLUSION

As we close this journey through the world of chair yoga and fitness for men over 40, it's important to reflect on the profound impact that these simple yet effective exercises can have on your life. Throughout this book, we've explored a variety of exercises designed to enhance balance, promote weight loss, improve mobility, increase flexibility, build core strength, prevent injuries, and better posture. Each exercise, from the gentle warm-ups to the more challenging poses, has been tailored to meet the unique needs of men in this age group.

The beauty of this approach lies in its simplicity and accessibility. Whether you're new to fitness or looking to adapt your routine to suit your changing body, the exercises in this book provide a safe and effective way to stay active and healthy. Regular practice can lead to significant improvements in your physical well-being, mental clarity, and overall quality of life.

Remember, the journey to better health is a personal one, and it's never too late to start. Be consistent with your practice, listen to your body, and make adjustments as needed. With dedication and patience, the benefits of these exercises will unfold, leading to a stronger, more flexible, and balanced you.

As you incorporate these exercises into your daily routine, embrace the changes and challenges they bring. Let this book be your guide to a healthier, more active, and balanced lifestyle. Here's to your health, strength, and vitality!

Thank you for reading

Thank you so much for choosing and reading my book! I appreciate you. Your support means the world to me. If you enjoyed your journey through the pages, I would be incredibly grateful if you could take a moment to leave a positive feedback on Amazon. Your feedback not only helps me grow as an author but also assists fellow readers in discovering this book. Thank you once again for being an amazing part of my writing journey!